STUDY GUIDE TO ACCOMPANY

W9-CEI-492

ESSENTIALS
of PHARMACOLOGY

for Health Occupations

6th Edition

STUDY GUIDE TO ACCOMPANY

ESSENTIALS of PHARMACOLOGY

for Health Occupations

6th Edition

Ruth Woodrow, RN, MA

Bruce J. Colbert, MS, RRT

David M. Smith, RPh, MS

DELMAR
CENGAGE Learning

Australia • Brazil • Japan • Korea • Mexico • Singapore • Spain • United Kingdom • United States

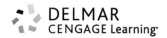
DELMAR
CENGAGE Learning·

Essentials of Pharmacology for Health Occupations, Sixth Edition
Ruth Woodrow, Bruce J. Colbert,
David M. Smith

Vice President, Career and Professional Editorial: Dave Garza

Director of Learning Solutions: Matthew Kane

Acquisitions Editor: Matthew Seeley

Managing Editor: Marah Bellegarde

Senior Product Manager: Debra Myette-Flis

Editorial Assistant: Samantha Zullo

Vice President, Career and Professional Marketing: Jennifer Baker

Executive Marketing Manager: Wendy Mapstone

Senior Marketing Manager: Kristin McNary

Marketing Coordinator: Scott Chrysler

Production Director: Carolyn S. Miller

Senior Content Project Manager: Kenneth McGrath

Senior Art Director: Jack Pendleton

Library of Congress Control Number: 2010926939

ISBN-13: 978-1-4354-8037-7

ISBN-10: 1-4354-8037-6

Delmar
5 Maxwell Drive
Clifton Park, NY 12065-2919
USA

Cengage Learning products are represented in Canada by Nelson Education, Ltd.

For your lifelong learning solutions, visit **delmar.cengage.com**

Visit our corporate website at **cengage.com**

Printed in the United States of America
7 8 9 10 11   19 18 17 16 15

CONTENTS

INTRODUCTION

Essentials of Pharmacology for Health Occupations, Sixth Edition, provides an extensive framework of drug information in a concise format. Drugs are organized by classifications and include their purpose, side effects, cautions, and interactions.

TO THE LEARNER

Each chapter in the study guide corresponds to the same chapter in the text. A variety of exercises are included to help reinforce the material you learned in the book. Types of exercises include Fill-in-the-Blank, Multiple Choice, Matching, and True or False. Part II chapters include case studies that encourage you to apply medication knowledge to clinical scenarios.

ESSENTIALS OF PHARMACOLOGY FOR HEALTH OCCUPATIONS, SIXTH EDITION, STUDYWARE™

Gain additional practice with the StudyWARE™ CD-ROM that offers an exciting way to enhance your learning of pharmacology. The quizzes and activities are an interactive and engaging way to reinforce the content in the book. Review the "*Essentials of Pharmacology for Health Occupations*, Sixth Edition, StudyWARE™" in your book for a detailed description of this component.

Introduction to Pharmacologic Principles

Consumer Safety and Drug Regulations

Fill-in-the-Blank

Fill in the blank for each of the following statements.

1. The law in reference to drug standards says that all preparations called by the same drug name must be of uniform _____, _____, and _____ no matter which pharmacy or which state the prescription for that drug is filled.

2. The Pure Food and Drug Act of 1906 established two references _____ _____ _____ (USP) and the _____ _____, which would specify the official U.S. standards for making every drug.

3. In 1970 a new department, the _____ _____ _____, was set up to enforce the Controlled Substances Act.

4. _____ and _____ health workers who may legally give medications include physicians, physician assistants, paramedics, medical office assistants, and practical, vocational, and registered nurses.

5. Dentists, physicians, physician assistants, veterinarians, nurse practitioners, and registered pharmacists may write prescriptions for their specific _____ of work within limitations.

6. Controlled drugs and those that cause dangerous health threats from side effects if taken incorrectly are ruled illegal to purchase without the use of a _____.

7. Numerous illegal _____ exist and operate to produce drugs within the United States today.

8. A health care practitioner in a doctor's office or clinic should _____ and _____ all prescription pads in the facility.

Multiple Choice

Circle the letter that best answers the question.

1. Which of these provisions was included as part of The Federal Food, Drug, and Cosmetic Act of 1938?

   A. All medication labels would be uniform in size
   B. All new products must be approved by the FDA before public release
   C. Established guidelines for each of the five schedules of controlled substances
   D. Established standards of effectiveness of medications

3

2. Which of the following acts declared that prescription and nonprescription drugs must be both safe and effective?

    A. Controlled Substance Act 1970
    B. Drug Enforcement Administration 1970
    C. Federal Food, Drug, and Cosmetic Act 1938
    D. Pure Food and Drug Act 1906

3. Each health care practitioner must be aware of regulations for controlled substances in their particular area because:

    A. Some states do not take part in these regulations.
    B. Some prescribers do not have to register to obtain a DEA number.
    C. Some prescribers only recognize Schedules C-I and C-II.
    D. Some states may have stricter schedules than the federal regulations.

4. Drug standards can best be described as:

    A. Established references for all drugs.
    B. Laws that enforce controlled substances.
    C. Rules set to assure consumers that they get what they pay for.
    D. Proof that the consumer will not have any adverse effects from the drug.

5. Which is these is a responsibility of The Food and Drug Administration?

    A. Supervising development of orphan drugs.
    B. Monitoring the need for changing the schedule of abused drugs.
    C. Inspecting plants where food, drugs, medical devices, or cosmetics are made.
    D. Enforcing laws against drug activities for illegal drug use.

6. The Drug Enforcement Administration has control over which of the following areas?

    A. Controlled substances
    B. Reviewing new drug applications and petitions for food additives
    C. Investigating and removing unsafe drugs from the market
    D. Monitoring sales of over the counter drugs

Matching

Match the guideline in Column A that should be followed by the health care practitioner when involved in dispensing medications with the rationale for that guideline in Column B.

COLUMN A	COLUMN B
_____ 1. Keep accurate records of controlled substance dispensed, received, or destroyed at your facility.	A. Prescription pads, with the physician's DEA registration number, are a possible source of fraud and drug tampering when forged and used illegally.
_____ 2. Keep a current drug reference book available at all times.	B. The health care practitioner involved in dispensing medications should be aware of any changes in safety standards and/or the scheduling of controlled substances.
_____ 3. When working in an office, maintain a professional rapport with the pharmaceutical representatives who leave drug samples.	C. The health care practitioner involved in dispensing medications should be able to readily identify substances that must be controlled.
_____ 4. Be responsible for keeping up to date with current news of the activities of the FDA and DEA.	D. Controlled substance record for the previous two years must be available at all times.

_____ 5. Conceal prescription pads at your office, clinic, or facility; keep pads in a designated location, out of public areas.

_____ 6. Keep controlled substances locked securely; double-locking is recommended.

_____ 7. Establish a working relationship with a local pharmacist.

E. This is an excellent resource for drug information.

F. This is an excellent resource for you when you are unsure of your legal responsibilities with drugs or have any uncertainties about drug therapy.

G. Placing controlled drugs in a locked safety box or placing a locked box in a cupboard that is locked will help prevent stealing and/or tampering with medications.

True or False

Circle T for true or F for false after reading each of the following statements.

1. T F Health care practitioners have an impact on the lives of others by appropriately or inappropriately responding to questions about medications, prescriptions, and drug therapy.

2. T F All drugs in the United States are made in federally approved laboratories.

3. T F In the market of illicit drugs, the lack of enforcement of drug standards is dangerous for the consumer.

4. T F The Pure Food and Drug Act of 1906 established the first government attempt to establish consumer protection in the manufacture of drugs and foods.

5. T F Controlled substances are arranged with the potentially most dangerous at level V and the least dangerous at level I.

6. T F A prescription for a C-II medication cannot be phoned in by an office health care practitioner.

7. T F Xanax is a schedule III medication and the prescription cannot be called in or faxed by a health care practitioner.

8. T F Controlled substance schedule numbers appear in a variety of drug information resources such as the Physician's Desk Reference, drug packages, and drug inserts.

9. T F The Drug Enforcement Administration (DEA) is solely concerned with controlled substances.

10. T F Using, dealing, and manufacturing of illegal drugs require the enforcement of the laws against drug activities by the Food and Drug Administration (FDA).

11. T F The Food and Drug Administration (FDA) may need to reassess and change its approval decision on a drug.

12. T F All herbal medicines and dietary supplements are safe.

CHAPTER 2

Drug Names and References

Fill-in-the-Blank

Fill in the blank for each of the following statements.

1. Drugs that affect the body in similar ways are recognized by groups and listed in the same _classification_.

2. For 17 years, from the time a company submits a new drug application to FDA for approval, that company has the exclusive right to _market_ the drug.

3. Pharmacology can be defined as the study of drugs and their origin, nature, properties, and effects on living _organism_.

4. It is the health care practitioner's responsibility to caution the layperson regarding the controversial and _care_ practices of "online prescribing" without ever having an evaluation in person by a physician, physician assistant, nurse practitioner, or dentist.

5. The health care practitioner should teach patients to read and _____ all ingredients on the label of over-the-counter medications before substituting them for prescription medications.

6. When a physician writes a prescription for a medication and prefers that the medication not be substituted with a generic form, the physician will indicate on the prescription "no _____" or DAW
(_____ _____ _____).

7. In the combination medications of Tylenol and codeine, the larger the number in the name, the greater the amount of controlled _____ present.

8. Damage to the kidneys, resulting in impaired kidney function, decreased urinary output, and renal failure is the result of _____.

9. An increased reaction to sunlight, with the danger of intense sunburn, is called _____.

10. A list of other drugs or foods that may alter the effect of the drug and usually should not be given during the same course of therapy would be noted under the heading _____ in a drug reference book.

11. "Usual _____" is a heading in a drug reference book that lists the amount of drug considered safe for administration and the route and frequency of administration.

12. "How Supplied" is a heading in a drug reference book that lists the available forms and _____ of a drug.

13. When using the Internet as a resource or reference for accurate drug information, care must be taken to identify and use only web sites that are supervised and _____, such as those under the auspices of government agencies or those sponsored by professional pharmacist groups.

14. Because it is difficult to know which of the many side effects are most likely to occur, some reference books underline or _____ the most common side effects.

15. When using the Internet as a reference, be wary of information from forums and _____, which are often sources of information that is not necessarily valid.

Multiple Choice

Circle the letter that best answers the question.

1. When researching drug information, a list of medical conditions or diseases for which the drug is meant to be used would be under which of the following headings?

   A. Cautions
   B. Actions
   C. Interactions
   D. Indications

2. Which of the following would describe *side effects* and *adverse reactions* listed in a drug information book?

   A. A technical description of the cellular and tissue changes that occur as a result of the drug
   B. A list of possible unpleasant or dangerous secondary effects other than the desired effect
   C. A list of conditions or types of patients that warrant close observation for specific side effects when given the drug
   D. A list of other drugs or food that may alter the effect of the drug and usually should not be given

3. Which of the following best describes *ototoxicity*, a side effect associated with antibiotics?

   A. Damage to the eighth cranial nerve that may be permanent or reversible, resulting in impaired hearing or tinnitus
   B. Damage to the kidneys resulting in impaired kidney function, decreased urinary output, and possibly renal failure
   C. Danger of intense sunburn due to an increased reaction to sunlight
   D. Danger of dehydration due to vomiting and diarrhea

4. Which of the following is specific information about the contraindications for a medication in a drug information book?

   A. A description of the cellular changes that occur as a result of the drug
   B. A list of medical diseases for which the drug is meant
   C. A possible unpleasant or dangerous secondary effect
   D. A list of conditions for which the drug should not be given

5. A *legend drug* is a:

   A. Drug on which the patent has expired.
   B. Drug with the same generic and chemical name.
   C. Prescription drug determined unsafe for over-the-counter purchase.
   D. Over-the-counter drug that many companies are producing.

6. The official name of a drug is the:

   A. Name by which a pharmaceutical company identifies its product.
   B. Description of the exact molecular formula of the drug.
   C. Name of the drug as it appears in the official reference.
   D. Common or general name by which most physicians refer to it.

7. Which of the following has the largest amount of codeine?

   A. Tylenol No. 1
   B. Tylenol No. 2
   C. Tylenol No. 3
   D. Tylenol No. 4

8. Birth control pills, cardiac drugs, hormones, and antibiotics are all examples of:

   A. Legend drugs.
   B. Over-the-counter medications.
   C. Controlled substances.
   D. Combination drugs.

9. When the drug reference describes *cautions*, it is referring to:

   A. A description of the cellular changes that occur as a result of the drug.
   B. A list of conditions or types of patients that warrant closer observation for specific side effects.
   C. A list of medical conditions or diseases for which the drug is meant to be used.
   D. A list of other drugs or foods that may alter the effect of the drug.

10. In order to avoid a drug error, the health care practitioner should do which of the following?

   A. Administer three Tylenol tablets when Tylenol No. 3 is ordered.
   B. Always check a reference before administering a medication with which you are not familiar.
   C. Consult the patient's chart for the history of allergies before a new medication is given.
   D. Identify any generic components of medications before administration.

Matching

Match the term in Column A with the definition in Column B.

COLUMN A	COLUMN B
_____ 1. Generic name	A. Prescription drug; determined unsafe for over-the-counter purchase because of possible harmful side effects if taken indiscriminately.
_____ 2. Controlled substance	B. The name by which a pharmaceutical company identifies its product. It is copyrighted and used exclusively by that company, and it can be distinguished from the generic name by its capitalized first letter.
_____ 3. Trade name	C. Common or general name assigned to a drug. It is differentiated from the trade name by its lowercase first letter; never capitalized.
_____ 4. Official name	D. No purchasing restrictions by the FDA.
_____ 5. Legend drug	E. Name of drug as it appears in the official reference, the *USP/NF*; generally the same as the generic name.
_____ 6. Over-the-counter drug	F. Drug restricted by prescription requirement because of the danger of addiction or abuse; indicated in references by schedule numbers C-I to C-V.
_____ 7. Chemical name	G. The exact molecular formula of the drug; usually long and very difficult to pronounce.

True or False

Circle T for true or F for false after reading each of the following statements.

1. T F A prototype is a drug that is a model example and typifies the characteristics of the drugs in the classification in which they are categorized.

2. T F Aspirin has a variety of therapeutic effects and is categorized under at least three classifications.

3. T F Tylenol No. 3 has a larger dosage of acetaminophen than Tylenol No. 2.

4. T F Specific provisions of *drug substitution* laws vary from state to state.

5. T F An advantage of the *Physician's Desk Reference (PDR)* is the easily identified nursing implications outlined for each drug.

6. T F Easy-to-read, practical guidelines for the patient are considered an advantage when using the *United States Pharmacopeia/Dispensing Information (USP/DI)* as a resource.

7. T F *AHFS Drug Information (American Health-System Formulary Service)* is arranged by classifications with a general statement about each classification at the beginning of each section.

8. T F Each health care practitioner must be aware of possible side effects prior to administering medications.

9. T F Trade name products are generally more expensive, although the basic active ingredients are the same as the generic.

10. T F The generic name will always appear with the first letter capitalized.

11. T F Benadryl must be used cautiously with patients who have a history of bronchial asthma.

12. T F Preparing and using drug cards reinforces learning and makes information easier and faster to locate.

Sources and Bodily Effects of Drugs

Fill-in-the-Blank

Fill in the blank for each of the following statements.

1. Any chemical substance ingested or applied on the body for the purpose of affecting body function is referred to as a _____.

2. Historically, _____ were the primary source of drugs, and bark, berries, leaves, resin from trees, and roots are still important drug sources.

3. Iron, sulfur, potassium, silver, and gold are examples of _____ used to prepare drugs.

4. When introduced into the body, all drugs cause cellular changes or drug actions that are followed by physiological changes, called _____ _____.

5. Medications contraindicated for lactating mothers have the ability to pass through the _____ _____ into the breast milk of the mother.

6. When drug compounds are produced from artificial rather than natural substances, the sources are called _____.

7. Drugs of a slightly acidic nature are absorbed well within the acidic _____ mucosa.

8. Drugs of an alkaline pH are absorbed better through the alkaline environment of the _____ _____.

9. Drug effects that reach widespread areas of the body are categorized as having a _____ effect.

10. The pituitary gland from _____ can be used to make a drug for the treatment of growth disorders.

11. A recent investigational drug called _____ (Cognex) was used to slow the progression of dementia in some patients with Alzheimer's disease and has been recalled because it produces liver toxicity.

12. An investigational drug developed in the 1990 that has been used to treat many different malignancies and in the management of AIDS-related Kaposi's sarcoma is called _____ (_____).

13. A new combination drug called Caduet combines Norvasc and Lipitor for simultaneous treatment of high _____ _____ and high _____.

14. Drug effects are generally categorized as _____ or _____.

15. A _____ effect is an increased effect of a drug demonstrated when repeated doses accumulate in the body that may build to a dangerous or toxic level.

16. The _____ route of drug administration is the easiest, but the effects are slower because of the time required for disintegration of drugs in the alimentary canal before absorption.

17. The _____ route of drug administration is the fastest because drugs enter the blood stream immediately.

18. The _____ route of drug administration with immediate effects can be quite dangerous if given in amounts recommended for other routes.

19. Getting an accurate drug history and clearly listing of _____ _____ is a critical function of the health care practitioner.

Multiple Choice

Circle the letter that best answers the question.

1. Which of the following best describes a local effect of a drug?

   A. Analgesic taken by mouth that provides general reduction in pain
   B. Phenergan suppository with broad absorption throughout the body with an antiemetic effect
   C. Acetaminophen suppository providing general reduction in fever
   D. Dibucaine ointment applied rectally, reducing hemorrhoidal pain

2. Discussion of the movement of medications from the blood stream into the tissues and fluids of the body is called:

   A. Absorption
   B. Distribution
   C. Metabolism
   D. Excretion

3. Which of the following best describes "selective distribution"?

   A. Substances high in lipid solubility quickly and easily absorbed through the stomach mucosa
   B. An increased effect of a drug when repeated doses accumulate in the body
   C. An affinity or attraction of a drug to a specific organ or cells
   D. A condition that results from exposure to a dangerous amount of a drug that is normally safe when given in a smaller amount

4. A patient with hepatic disease may exhibit toxic (poisonous) effects of a drug due to altered metabolism because the drug is not:

   A. being properly broken down by the inefficient liver.
   B. being eliminated through the lungs or through perspiration.
   C. able to pass the blood-brain barrier.
   D. able to pass through the placental barrier.

5. An example of drugs that have selective distribution is the attraction of amphetamines to the:

   A. Liver
   B. Kidneys
   C. Cerebrospinal fluid
   D. Stomach

6. The goal of drug therapy is to give just enough of the drug to cause which of these effects?

   A. Therapeutic
   B. Toxic
   C. Placebo
   D. Lethal

7. When administering the cardiac drug digoxin, the health care practitioner should recognize that if the patient's circulation and renal function are inadequate, which of these cumulative effects is produced?

   A. An episode of a rapid heart rate
   B. Dilated pupils
   C. Jaundiced skin
   D. Dangerously low heart rate

8. Because children have a lower threshold of response and react more rapidly and sometimes in unexpected ways which of these actions is necessary?

   A. Frequent assessment
   B. Administering medications only in the hospital
   C. Prescribing a higher dose of medication
   D. Withholding most medications

9. When are placebos are most often used in health care?

   A. With patients who have heart disease.
   B. For patients participating in a blind study experiment.
   C. For patients who are over 65 years of age.
   D. With patients who have inadequate circulation and renal function.

10. Synergism refers to the:

   A. Action of two drugs in which one prolongs or multiplies the effect of the other.
   B. Opposing action of two drugs in which one decreases or cancels out the effect of the other.
   C. Administration of two or more medications at one time.
   D. Action of two drugs working together in which one helps the other simultaneously for an effect that neither could produce alone.

11. Which of the following describes an undesirable synergism?

   A. Sedatives and barbiturates given in combination, resulting in depression of the central nervous system
   B. Promethazine and meperidine given in combination, resulting in more effective pain relief
   C. Tagamet and Tofranil given in combination, potentiating the antisecretory effect
   D. Antacids taken at the same time as tetracycline, altering pH and preventing the absorption of tetracycline

12. The physician's choice of a particular route of medication administration has the greatest significance for

   A. How rapidly or slowly the results are desired
   B. Therapeutic effectiveness
   C. Where the drug is absorbed
   D. Cost of the drug

13. Parenteral routes include:

   A. Rectal
   B. Nasogastric
   C. Sublingual
   D. Oral

14. When giving a medication to a patient for the first time, the health care practitioner should assess for a hypersensitivity response in patients who

   A. Complain of nausea from a previous medication
   B. Have history of known allergies
   C. Complain of diarrhea from a previous medication
   D. Take more than one medication

15. Persons who have had an anaphylactic reaction to a substance should always:

   A. Take the medication on an empty stomach.
   B. Be prepared to lie down for at least 30 minutes after taking medications.
   C. Wear a Medic-Alert tag or bracelet to identify the date of the previous reaction.
   D. Wear a Medic-Alert tag or bracelet to identify the substance to which they are extremely allergic.

16. Treatment for anaphylactic reaction may include CPR and which of the following medications?

   A. Narcan, Tagamet, and Phenergan
   B. Digoxin, Norvasc, and Lipitor
   C. Epinephrine, a corticosteroid, and an antihistamine
   D. An amphetamine and an antidepressant

Matching A

Match the dosage description in Column A with the definition in Column B.

COLUMN A	COLUMN B
_____ 1. Minimal dose	A. Dose required to keep the drug blood level at a steady state in order to maintain the desired effect
_____ 2. Maximum dose	B. Dose that is customarily given (average adult dose based on body weight of 150 lb), adjusted according to variations from the norm
_____ 3. Loading dose	C. Initial high dose used to quickly elevate the level of drug in the blood (often followed by a series of lower maintenance doses)
_____ 4. Maintenance dose	D. Smallest amount of drug that will produce a therapeutic effect
_____ 5. Toxic dose	E. Dose that causes death
_____ 6. Lethal dose	F. Largest amount of a drug that will produce a desired effect without producing symptoms of toxicity
_____ 7. Therapeutic dose	G. Amount of a drug that will produce harmful side effects or symptoms of poisoning

Matching B

Match the terms describing unexpected responses to drugs in Column A with the description of the term in Column B.

COLUMN A	COLUMN B
_____ 1. Teratogenic	A. Severe hypersensitivity response, possibly requiring CPR; may be fatal allergic reaction
_____ 2. Idiosyncrasy	B. Immune response to a drug that may be of varying degrees
_____ 3. Paradoxical	C. Effect from maternal drug administration that causes the development of physical defects in a fetus
_____ 4. Tolerance	D. Acquired need for a drug that may produce psychological and/or physical symptoms of withdrawal when the drug is discontinued
_____ 5. Dependence	E. Unique, unusual response to a drug
_____ 6. Hypersensitivity	F. Decreased response to a drug that develops after repeated doses are given
_____ 7. Anaphylactic reaction	G. Opposite effect from the drug that was expected

True or False

Circle T for true or F for false after reading each of the following statements.

1. T F Substances low in lipid solubility are absorbed best when given by a means other than the GI tract.

2. T F Oral elixir medications administered to infants are always absorbed better if given with or just after infant formula.

3. T F If a fast drug effect is desired, an empty stomach will facilitate quicker absorption.

4. T F During biotransformation in the liver, a drug is broken down and altered to more water-soluble by-products so that it may be more easily excreted by the kidneys.

5. T F Digoxin is a cardiac drug that must be given cautiously because of its cumulative effect, called "digoxin toxicity."

6. T F Metabolism and excretion are more rapid in older adults, and therefore attention must be paid to possible cumulative effects.

7. T   F   Many drug dosages are calculated on the basis of the patient's weight.

8. T   F   There are few individual variations in sensitivity to drugs.

9. T   F   Attention must be paid to the variable of gender when administering medications because the ratio of fat per body mass differs in men and women.

10. T   F   A placebo is a smaller amount of the medication with extra saline solution added.

11. T   F   Attitudes toward medicines can be influenced positively or negatively by cultural or religious beliefs.

12. T   F   The health care practitioner administering or assisting with the administration of medications must recognize that his or her attitude regarding a medication may be picked up by the patient and indirectly may affect the response the drug.

13. T   F   An example of a desirable antagonism is a narcotic antagonist that saves lives from drug overdoses by canceling out the effect of narcotics.

14. T   F   The intramuscular route is the best route for emergencies because of the speed of action.

15. T   F   Parenteral routes are the choice when patients can take nothing by mouth.

16. T   F   The transdermal route of drug administration allows for slower consistent drug administration over time.

17. T   F   The inhalation route of drug administration is often more effective and easier for the patient.

Case Study

Greg Wilson, a 65-year-old man, is diagnosed with pneumonia. He has a history of congestive heart failure. His physician has ordered an antibiotic for the pneumonia and he takes digoxin every day.

1. As the health care provider, which of the following questions would you ask before administering his antibiotic?

   A. "How long have you been taking the heart pill?"
   B. "Have you ever had an allergic reaction to an antibiotic?"
   C. "What is the best time of day for you to take the medications?"
   D. "How tall are you?"

2. Why is the first dose of the antibiotic twice as much as the maintenance doses?

   A. To assess if the medication will cause paradoxical effects.
   B. The minimum dose is the smallest dose that can be given.
   C. The loading dose is used to quickly elevate the level of the antibiotic in the blood.
   D. Psychological dependence on the drug will be decreased if a larger dose is given first.

3. While Greg is in the hospital he will receive the antibiotic intravenously. The rationale for this is:

   A. The medication enters the blood stream immediately.
   B. The cost of intravenous medications is cheaper.
   C. If taken orally, the medication has an unpleasant taste.
   D. The medication is less toxic when administered intravenously.

4. While Greg is in the hospital he has blood drawn for a digoxin level. What symptoms would Greg likely exhibit if his digoxin level was higher than the therapeutic level?

   A. High cholesterol levels
   B. Low hemoglobin levels
   C. Faster heart rate
   D. Slower heart rate

5. Which of the following variables may slow the metabolism and excretion of Greg's medications and possibly cause a cumulative effect?

   A. Gender
   B. Psychological state
   C. Age
   D. Time of year

CHAPTER 4

Medication Preparations and Supplies

Fill-in-the-Blank

Fill in the blank for each of the following statements.

1. _Parenteral_ refers to any route not involving the GI tract, including injection, topical, and inhalation routes.

2. A tablet with a special coating that resists disintegration by gastric juices due to the outside layer is called an _enteric_-_coated_ tablet.

3. A liquid form of medication that must be shaken well before administration because drug particles settle at the bottom of the bottle is called a _suspension_.

4. Dilution of a powder form of medication in a sterile solution is called _____ of a drug.

5. The parenteral route in which drugs are injected into the subarachnoid space is called _____.

6. A rectal drug form with the drug suspended in a substance such as cocoa butter that melts at body temperature is called a _suppository_.

7. The most common classifications of drugs given rectally include sedatives, antipyretics, and _antiemetics_.

8. Dermal patches vary in size, shape, and color and are used for management of conditions as varied as prevention of angina and motion sickness, and management of chronic _pain_.

9. The health care provider may be asked to instill drugs in sterile liquids by drops into the eye, _ear_, and _nose_.

10. A sterile semisolid preparation, often antibiotic in nature, for ophthalmic use only is called an _____ _____.

11. Patients with moderate to severe asthma rely on the use of _____ to keep their airways open by inhaling the mist of a bronchodilator.

12. The Occupational Safety and Health Administration (OSHA) mandated efforts to reduce the risk of _____-_____ injuries by using safety needles with a protective sheath that covers the needle automatically immediately after administration or one that retracts into the syringe on administration.

Multiple Choice

Circle the letter that best answers the questions.

1. Tuberculin skin tests (PPD) are administered through which route?

   A. IV piggyback
   B. Intramuscular
   C. Epidural
   D. Intradermal

2. What drug form is designed to deliver a dose of drug over an extended period of time?

   A. Lozenge
   B. Enteric-coated tablet
   C. Sustained-release capsule
   D. Enema solution

3. Which of the following is an advantage of using the transdermal delivery system?

   A. Blood level of medication peaks at two-hour intervals.
   B. It applies easily, with no discomfort or undesirable taste.
   C. Some drugs are effective for up to a year and are used for clients with skin disorders.
   D. The double chamber may be pulled apart to add drug powder to soft foods or beverages.

4. Only physicians can administer medications by which of these parenteral routes?

   A. Intraspinal
   B. Intradermal
   C. Intramuscular
   D. Intravenous

5. The oral route of medication administration is the route of choice for most patients because it is

   A. Effective for treatment of emergencies
   B. Tolerated by all patients who are NPO
   C. Provides the most rapid absorption rate and drug effect
   D. Cheapest and easiest route

6. Which of the following best describes an IV push intravenous injection?

   A. A small volume of drug injected through a syringe and needle into a peripheral saline lock (PRN adapter)
   B. A drug diluted in a moderate volume of fluid for intermittent infusion at specified intervals
   C. A large volume of fluids that infuse continuously into a vein with or without medication added
   D. A drug injected into a catheter that has been placed by an anesthesiologist in the epidural space of the spinal canal

7. Of the following, which best describes correctly how to administer an intradermal injection?

   A. Using a standard hypodermic syringe, inject 0.5–1 mL of the drug at a 90 degree angle with the bevel down.
   B. Using a TB syringe, inject 0.1–0.2 mL of the drug at a 15 degree angle with the bevel of the needle up just under the skin.
   C. Using a standard U-100 insulin syringe, inject 1–2 mL of the drug at a 45-degree angle in the dermis.
   D. Using a PRN adapter attached to a vein, inject by pushing directly into vein.

8. A skin patch containing drug molecules that can be absorbed through the skin to promote a consistent blood level between application times describes which of these applications?

   A. Liniment
   B. Ointment
   C. Dermal patch
   D. Lotion

9. Which of the following medications may be delivered through nebulization by the respiratory therapist in an acute care setting?

    A. Nitroglycerin
    B. Duragesic
    C. Bronchodilator
    D. Sedative

10. The number that represents the diameter of the needle lumen and ranges from 18 to 27 is called the

    A. Calibration
    B. Gauge
    C. Suspension
    D. Ampule

11. Medication that is absorbed via the mucosa under the tongue is called a

    A. Buccal tablet
    B. Timed-release capsule
    C. Sublingual tablet
    D. Enteric-coated tablet

12. What term describes a glass container sealed at the top by a rubber stopper containing 1–2 mL of sterile solution that is removed to provide a single dose of medication?

    A. Ampule
    B. Mortar
    C. Pestle
    D. Unit-dose vial

13. Implantable devices are used to deliver which of these types of medications?

    A. Insulin
    B. Antibiotics
    C. Vitamins
    D. Antipyretics

14. Intravenous administration provides the fastest action of a medication. What is the second fastest route of drug administration?

    A. Intramuscular
    B. Inhalation
    C. Intradermal
    D. Subcutaneous

Matching

Match the definition or abbreviation in Column A with the correct term in Column B.

COLUMN A	COLUMN B
_____ 1. Liquid drug that forms with alcohol base	A. Tablet
_____ 2. Per os	B. Syrup
_____ 3. Tablet that resists disintegration by gastric juices	C. Drop
_____ 4. Disk of compressed drug	D. Lozenge
_____ 5. Indicated for local soothing effect on the throat or mouth	E. Emulsion
_____ 6. Liquid drug that contains oils and fats in water	F. Intracardiac injection
_____ 7. Sweetened, flavored liquid drug form	G. Oral

(Matching continued on next page)

COLUMN A **(continued)**	**COLUMN B** **(continued)**

_____ 8. GTT

H. Enteric-coated tablet

_____ 9. Liquid drug in which drug particles settle to the bottom of the bottle

I. Vaginal cream

_____ 10. Medication injected directly into the heart

J. Elixir

_____ 11. The type of preparation in which the drug is supplied

K. Suspension

_____ 12. Antibiotic or antifungal cream inserted vaginally with a special applicator

L. Douche solution

_____ 13. Sterile antiseptic solution and sterile water used to irrigate the vaginal canal

M. Drug form

True or False

Circle T for true or F for false after reading each of the following statements.

1. T   F   When discussing routes for medications, "Parenteral" refers to any route involving the GI tract.

2. T   F   When a tablet is scored, this indicates that there is even distribution of the drug in halves or quarters if it is broken on the scored lines.

3. T   F   In order for the enteric-coated tablet to be effective against the medication irritating the stomach, the coating must never be destroyed by chewing or crushing before administration.

4. T   F   Timed-release capsules work most effectively when taken with applesauce or ice cream after being opened and sprinkled on the food.

5. T   F   The health care provider should always teach patients to keep elixirs tightly capped.

6. T   F   A subcutaneous injection is injected into the fatty layer of tissue below the skin using a 45-degree angle or a 90-degree angle.

7. T   F   Unit-dose vials contain up to 50 mL of solution and may be repeatedly entered through the rubber stopper to remove a portion of the medication.

8. T   F   An ampule must be broken at the neck to obtain the single dose of sterile solution for injection.

9. T   F   Before administration of insulin, the dosage should always be double-checked by two caregivers.

10. T   F   The advantage of nitroglycerin ointment and/or dermal patch is their ability to prevent angina by the slow, consistent release of the drug over a period of time.

11. T   F   The subcutaneous route, rather than the IM route, is the route of choice when medications should be absorbed more rapidly.

12. T   F   IV push medications are available for immediate absorption and availability to major organs, which make this route a dangerous one.

13. T   F   Medications administered intradermally cause a greater reaction locally than systemically.

14. T   F   The mortar and pestle are used for mixing liquid medications before administration.

15. T   F   Insulin can be measured in an insulin syringe or a TB syringe.

16. T   F   The terms *drug form* and *drug preparation* are synonymous.

CHAPTER 5

Abbreviations and Systems of Measurement

Fill-in-the-Blank

Fill in the blank for each of the following statements.

1. The first responsibility of the health care practitioner when preparing medication for administration is _____ of the medication order.

2. When in doubt about the interpretation of a medication order always question the meaning, never _____.

3. Medication orders must always be written and signed by a _____.

4. During an emergency the health care practitioner may be given a _____ order by the physician, which will be signed by the physician after the emergency.

5. When receiving a verbal order the health care practitioner's responsibility is to _____ _____ the name of the medication and the amount to the physician before administration.

6. When a verbal order is followed and the medication is administered it is the responsibility of the health care practitioner to document the medication, amount, and _____ of administration.

7. The medical assistant or nurse who will be calling in a prescription for the physician should repeat the name of the drug, _____, frequency, and route back to the physician as the order is written down.

8. The abbreviation PCA means _____ _____ _____.

9. A written prescription for a controlled substance reads "2 tabs q4h," which means: 2 _____ every 4 _____.

10. The abbreviation "Fe" represents the term _____.

11. The apothecary system of measuring solids includes drams, ounces, and _____.

12. One gram is equal to _____ mg and _____ gr.

Multiple Choice

Circle the letter that best answers the question.

1. In most states the physician must sign all verbal and telephone orders within how many hours?

   A. 8
   B. 12
   C. 24
   D. 36

2. Which of the following is the correct documentation when receiving a telephone order?

   A. Doctor Jones nurse called @ 1600 and said to give Mr. Cavis a sleeping pill at bedtime. D. Hope CMA
   B. Ambien 10 mg. P.O. @ H.S., VO Dr. S. Jones, per Pat White CMA @ 1600. D. Hope CMA
   C. Lasix 40 mg. PO this a.m. for Mr. Cavis, room 6240, TO Dr. S. Jones, per Pat White CMA @ 1600.
      D. Hope CMA
   D. Give the patient in 6240 Lasix 40 mg. tomorrow morning, Dr. Jones per phone order. Hope CMA

3. Which of the following is an appropriate abbreviation for grain?

   A. g
   B. GM
   C. gtt
   D. gr

4. Which of the following is the correct interpretation of D5W with 20 mEq of KCL/L?

   A. Dextrose five percent in water with twenty milliequivalents of potassium chloride per liter
   B. Dextrose and water with twenty milligrams of potassium and normal saline mixed in each liter
   C. Distilled water with twenty micrograms of potassium chloride per pound
   D. Double strength dextrose and water with twenty millimeters of sodium chloride

5. When the physician orders a medication by NEB, the health care practitioner knows this refers to:

   A. Normal elixir base
   B. Nothing by mouth
   C. Administer by nebulizer
   D. Administer by nasogastric tube

6. Which of these measurements are used for measuring solid weights in the metric system?

   A. Gram and milligram
   B. Liter and milliliter
   C. Minim and ounce
   D. Grain and dram

7. What is the metric equivalent of 1/2 grain?

   A. 500 milligrams
   B. 30 milligrams
   C. 0.5 gram
   D. 0.3 gram

8. 2 kg is equal to:

   A. 0.453592 pound
   B. 0.55555 pound
   C. 2.2 pounds
   D. 4.4 pounds

9. One teaspoon of a medication is equivalent to how many milliliters?

   A. 1 mL
   B. 5 mL
   C. 15 mL
   D. 30 mL

10. One thousand milliliters is equal to how many ounces?

    A. 8
    B. 16
    C. 24
    D. 32

Matching

Match the definition or abbreviation in Column A with the correct term in Column B.

	COLUMN A	COLUMN B
_____	1. Before meals	A. TID
_____	2. Twice a day	B. D5W
_____	3. Centimeter	C. RL
_____	4. Discontinue	D. Stat
_____	5. Dextrose 5% in water	E. OTC
_____	6. Extended release	F. SR
_____	7. Grain	G. Gtt
_____	8. Drop	H. ER
_____	9. Keep vein open	I. KVO
_____	10. Pound	J. BID
_____	11. Milliequivalent	K. Gr
_____	12. Microgram	L. Cm
_____	13. Sodium chloride	M. Lb
_____	14. Nothing by mouth	N. Ac
_____	15. Normal saline (sodium chloride, 0.9%)	O. mEq
_____	16. Over the counter	P. DC
_____	17. Ounce	Q. Mcg
_____	18. After meals	R. Oz
_____	19. As desired	S. NS
_____	20. Whenever necessary	T. Pc
_____	21. Ringer's lactate	U. PRN
_____	22. Sustained release	V. NaCl
_____	23. Immediately	W. ad lib
_____	24. Three times a day	X. NPO

True or False

Circle T for true or F for false after reading each of the following statements.

1. T F Regulations vary from state to state regarding phone orders concerning who can call in an order, who can receive an order, and the time frame for the physician's signature.

2. T F There should never be a blank space on a written prescription in the area asking for number of refills.

3. T F In order to avoid errors in dosage administration, periods should be placed after each medical abbreviation.

4. T F It is the responsibility of any health care practitioner dealing with the administration of medications in any health care setting to memorize the common abbreviations and symbols for medication orders.

5. T F The health care provider should teach patients to estimate or guess when they are unsure about the dosage of a medication.

6. T   F   One safety practice related to abbreviations and systems of measurement is the avoidance of periods with all medical abbreviations in order to avoid being mistaken as the number 1.

7. T   F   The abbreviation "IN" refers to intranasal but should not be used because it is on the Error-Prone list of abbreviations due to being mistaken as "IM" or "IV."

8. T   F   The household system of liquid measurement includes the minim, fluid dram, grain, and pound.

9. T   F   The metric system was invented by the French and is the international standard for weights and measures.

10. T   F   The health care practitioner teaching the patient and family about administering an elixir should instruct them to use a household teaspoon to measure all liquid medications.

11. T   F   Equipment most commonly used for measuring medications includes the medicine cup and various syringes calibrated in milliliters and/or minims.

12. T   F   One measuring cup in the household system can be converted to 4 oz in the apothecary system and 100 mL in the metric system.

13. T   F   Medications ordered in the apothecary measurement of grains can be converted to the metric system in grams or milligrams.

14. T   F   One tablespoon is equal to 30 mL and equal to 1 oz in liquid medications.

15. T   F   Medication ordered as 1/150 gr is equivalent to 0.4 mg.

16. T   F   Some states require that the quantity of a drug prescribed must be written in both text and numerical formats.

Safe Dosage Preparation

Fill-in-the-Blank

Fill in the blank for each of the following statements.

1. It is the responsibility of the health care practitioner to be absolutely certain that the medication administered is exactly as ___prescribe___ by the physician and is also an appropriate ___dose___ for that particular patient.

2. Medications dispensed by the pharmacist in _____-_____ form are prepackaged in a separate packet, vial, or prefilled syringe for each individual dose of a medicine.

3. Much of the mixing and measuring of medications is now completed by the pharmacist; however, the person administering medications must understand the preparation of dosages in order to ensure ___accuracy___.

4. Because a misplaced decimal point could cause a patient ___fatality (death)___, there is no margin of error in administration of medications.

5. Safe dosage preparation requires a working knowledge of basic arithmetic and meticulous care with all ___calculations___.

6. The first basic step in safe dosage preparation is to check whether all measures are in the same ___system___.

7. The second basic step in safe dosage preparation is to complete the necessary calculations by writing the problem in equation form using the appropriate ___formula___ and labeling all parts.

8. The third basic step in safe dosage preparation after completing necessary calculations is to check the accuracy of your answer for ___reasonableness___ and have someone verify your calculations.

9. A ratio describes a ___relationship___ between two numbers.

10. A proportion consists of two ___ratio___ that are equal.

11. When using the ratio and proportion method of calculation, the terms of each ratio must be in the same ___system (ml, mg)___.

12. To solve a problem with the ratio and proportion method, set up the formula with the known terms on the left and the ___desire___ terms on the right.

13. When solving the calculation using ratio and proportion, first verify that all measures are in the same ___system___.

14. When solving the calculation using ratio and proportion, it is important to label all ___terms___.

15. In neonates, renal function and some enzyme ___system___ needed for drug absorption and metabolism are not fully developed.

16. In neonates the total body water makes up a greater percentage of body weight than in children and adults, which affects drug ___absorption___.

23

17. When calculating appropriate dosages for children as well as adults, the health care provider must take into consideration variables such as age, weight, gender, and metabolic, psychological, or _pathological_ conditions.

18. When preparing drug dosages for children, it is important to always refer to recommended _dosages_ as listed in the drug insert or in a current drug reference.

19. Recommended dosages for children are often expressed in the drug reference as a number of milligrams per unit of _body_ _weight_, per unit of time.

20. Recommended dosages for children are derived from data obtained in clinical _trials_ utilizing sick children.

21. As a health care provider administering medications, it is your duty and _legal_ responsibility to be sure that the drugs you administer are safe.

22. Always _question_ an order if you have difficulty interpreting the spelling of a drug name or the number used for the dosage or the dosage seems inappropriate.

Multiple Choice

Circle the letter that best answers the question.

1. The order reads atropine sulfate 0.4 mg IM stat; available vials are labeled atropine sulfate 1 mg/mL. Using basic calculation, how much medication would be given?

   A. 0.4 mL
   B. 0.6 mL
   C. 1 mL
   D. 1.5 mL

2. When preparing to administer medications to the neonate, the health care practitioner must consider that the neonate's renal function and some enzyme systems are not fully developed and this affects a drug's:

   A. Route of ingestion.
   B. Selective distribution.
   C. Absorption and metabolism.
   D. Passage through the placental barrier.

3. Drug absorption in the neonate is affected by:

   A. The permeability of the blood-brain barrier.
   B. The neonate's gender
   C. The placental barrier.
   D. The father's blood type.

4. When a health care provider is using the basic calculation method to obtain correct medication dosage, which of these answers should be questioned?

   A. if it is less than ½ tab.
   B. if it is more than 1 tablet.
   C. if a subcutaneous injection if it is more than 1/mL.
   D. if the IM injection dosage is less than 1 mL.

5. The order reads: Administer Rocephin 150 mg IM every 12 hours. On hand is Rocephin 1g/10 mL. Using the basic calculation method, what is the first step the health care practitioner should take?

   A. Check for reasonableness.
   B. Use the formula and label all parts.
   C. Estimate the dosage and administer.
   D. Convert grams to milligrams.

6. The order reads: Administer Rocephin 150 mg IM every 12 hours. On hand is Rocephin 1g/10 mL. Using the basic calculation method, what is the second step the health care practitioner should take?

    A. Convert grams to milligrams.
    B. Use the formula and label all parts.
    C. Estimate the dosage and administer.
    D. Check for reasonableness.

7. The order reads: Administer Rocephin 150 mg IM every 12 hours. On hand is Rocephin 1g/10 mL. Using the basic calculation method, what is the third step the health care practitioner should take?

    A. Estimate the dosage and administer.
    B. Convert grams to milligrams.
    C. Check for reasonableness.
    D. Use the formula and label all parts.

8. The order reads: Administer Rocephin 150 mg IM every 12 hours. On hand is Rocephin 1g/10 mL. Using the basic calculation method, what amount of medication will the health care practitioner administer?

    A. 2.5 mL
    B. 1.5 mL
    C. 1 mL
    D. 0.5 mL

9. The order reads: Administer Tylenol 650 mg every 4 hours PRN. On hand is Tylenol 325 mg scored tablets. Using the basic calculation method, what amount of medication will the health care practitioner give?

    A. ½ tablet
    B. 1 tablet
    C. 1½ tablet
    D. 2 tablets

10. The order reads: Administer Phenergan 12.5 mg PO every 6 hours: On hand is Phenergan 25 mg scored tablets. Using the basic calculation method, what amount of medication will the health care practitioner give?

    A. 2 tablets
    B. 1½ tablets
    C. 1 tablet
    D. ½ tablet

11. To solve a problem with the ratio and proportion method, set up the formula with the known terms on the left and what terms on the right?

    A. The system measurement involved.
    B. The desired and unknown terms.
    C. The estimated answer.
    D. All terms labeled.

12. To solve a problem with the ratio and proportion method, multiply the two outer terms called the:

    A. Means.
    B. Extremes.
    C. Variables.
    D. Quantities.

13. To solve a problem with the ratio and proportion method, multiply the two inner terms called the:

    A. Means.
    B. Extremes.
    C. Variables.
    D. Quantities.

14. The order reads: Morphine sulfate 1/6 grain IM for pain: On hand is morphine sulfate 10 mg/mL. Using the ratio and proportion method, what is the first step the health care practitioner should take?

    A. Label all terms.
    B. Verify that the measures are in the same system.
    C. Set up the problem as a proportion.
    D. Verify the calculation.

15. The order reads: Morphine sulfate 1/6 grain IM for pain: On hand is morphine sulfate 10 mg/mL. If the equivalent of 1/6 grain is unknown, what would the health care practitioner do next?

    A. Use the formula and label all parts.
    B. Calculate the equivalent using the ratio and proportion method.
    C. Estimate the equivalent and administer.
    D. Check the answer for reasonableness.

16. The physician's order reads: Administer morphine 1/6 grain IM for pain to a pediatric patient. The health care practitioner is not familiar with the dosage for this child. What action should be taken first?

    A. Call the physician.
    B. Call the pharmacist.
    C. Look up the medication in a current drug reference.
    D. Administer the medication to the child.

17. The physician's order reads: Administer morphine 1/6 grain IM for pain. How many milligrams is 1/6 grain?

    A. 10
    B. 15
    C. 30
    D. 60

18. The physician's order reads: Administer morphine 1/6 grain IM for pain: On hand is morphine 10 mg/mL. Using the ratio and proportion method, how much medication should the health care practitioner administer?

    A. 0.5 mL
    B. 0.75 mL
    C. 1 mL
    D. 1.5 mL

19. The physician's order reads: Atropine sulfate 1/150 grain IM pre-operatively. How many mg is 1/150 grain?

    A. 0.4 mg
    B. 0.8 mg
    C. 1 mg
    D. 6 mg

20. The physician's order reads: Atropine sulfate 1/150 grain IM pre-operatively: On hand is atropine sulfate 1 mg/mL. Using the ratio and proportion method, how much atropine sulfate should the health care practitioner administer?

    A. 1 mL
    B. 0.8 mL
    C. 0.6 mL
    D. 0.4 mL

Matching

Match the calculation problem in Column A with the solution in Column B.
Column A Calculation Problems

COLUMN A	COLUMN B
_____ 1. 50 mg : 5 mL = 150 mg : X mL	A. 0.25 gm
_____ 2. 1 gm : 1000 mg = 0.35g : X mg	B. 68.2 kg
_____ 3. Give 500 mg tablets 4 times daily; on hand 250 mg tablets. Administer _X_tablets over 24 hours	C. 5 mL
_____ 4. 100 mg : 10 cc = 25 mg : X cc	D. 350 mg
_____ 5. 150 lb = X kg	E. 2.5 mL
_____ 6. Give 50 mg of medication now; on hand 25 mg capsules. Administer X capsules	F. 2 capsules
_____ 7. 250 mg = X gm	G. 8 tablets
_____ 8. Give 50 mg of liquid medication; on hand is 10mg/mL. Give X mL	H. 15 mL

True or False

Circle T for true or F for false after reading each of the following statements.

1. T F On occasion the dosage ordered differs from the dose on hand, making it necessary that the correct dosage be calculated.

2. T F There is no margin of error in administration of medications because it only takes a small error in arithmetic to seriously harm a patient.

3. T F Children are miniature adults and therefore the dosage can merely be divided and given to a child.

4. T F Neonates' blood-brain barrier is less permeable and more medication is needed even though the weight is low.

5. T F Digoxin is a cardiac drug that must be given cautiously because of its cumulative effect called digoxin toxicity.

6. T F Metabolism and excretion are more rapid in the older adult and, therefore, attention must be paid to possible cumulative effects.

7. T F Many drug dosages are calculated on the basis of the patient's weight.

8. T F Dehydration or electrolyte imbalance can affect assimilation of drugs and interfere with therapeutic effect.

9. T F Any older adult person taking many drugs is at risk for potentially lethal interactions.

10. T F In order to prevent medication errors, always place a decimal point and zero after writing a whole number.

11. T F If a medication error results in legal action, the health care provider could be held accountable, even though the order was written incorrectly.

12. T F The health care practitioner administering medications to children can check the appropriateness of the dose by applying *Clark's Rule*.

CHAPTER 7

Responsibilities and Principles of Drug Administration

Fill-in-the-Blank

Fill in the blank for each of the following statements.

1. Responsibility for safe administration of medications requires that the health care practitioner be familiar with every medication _____ administration.

2. Documentation on the patient's record is always _____ for all medications given.

3. Meticulous care in _____ and administration of medications reduces the chances of error.

4. When a medication error occurs, the health care practitioner is _____ required to complete an incident report.

5. Health care practitioners have a responsibility to provide quality care and provide for patient _____ at all times.

6. A major responsibility of the health care practitioner is to provide the patient and family with necessary _____ about the medications, side effects, and precautions prescribed for the patient.

7. The challenge of *"First do no harm"* includes _____ of medication errors and also _____ errors so that corrective steps can be taken.

8. As a part of the *"First do no harm"* the U.S. Pharmacopoeia (USP) has established a program called Medication _____ _____ (MER).

9. Confusion over the _____ of drug names, either written or spoken, accounts for approximately one-quarter of all error reports to the MER.

10. It is essential to safe administration of medications that health care practitioners always wash hands before _____ of medicines.

11. One of the responsibilities of the health care provider in safe administration of medications is to have adequate, up-to-date information about _____ medications administered.

12. Two major responsibilities of the health care provider in drug administration are _____ in delivery of the medication accurately, in the best interests of the patients, with adequate _____.

13. The health care provider administering drugs is responsible to provide education to the patient and family about why, when, and _____ their medications are to be taken.

14. The goal in drug administration is to maximize the effectiveness of the drug with the least _____ to the patient.

15. Teaching the patient and family about medications administration includes providing both verbal and _____ instructions.

16. Administration of medications by the health care provider carries moral, legal, and _____ responsibilities.

17. The health care practitioner should be especially careful when the dose of a medication is expressed in decimals or _____.

18. The health care practitioner should always _____ the dosage of a drug if less than 1 tablet or more than 1 tablet is required.

19. The health care practitioner should remember that the action of any drug is influenced by the patient's condition, metabolism, age, gender, psychological state, and _____.

20. The health care provider is responsible for reporting the results of careful _____ and observations to ensure the right dosage is prescribed for each patient.

21. Some medications need to be maintained at a specific level in the blood and are therefore prescribed at regular _____ around the clock (e.g., every 4 hours, every 8 hours).

22. If the physician does not prescribe a specific time for administration of a medication, the health care practitioner arranges an appropriate _____, taking into consideration the purpose, action, and side effects of the medication.

23. Health care practitioners administering medications have the right and responsibility to question the appropriateness of a route based on observation and _____ of the patient's condition.

24. Each medication given by the health care practitioner must be recorded on the patient's record, along with the dose, time, route and _____ of injections.

25. The responsibility of documentation for the health care practitioner administering medications includes the recording of any _____ _____ on the special control substances record.

26. The health care practitioner can help the FDA better monitor product safety and take swift action to protect patients and health care practitioners by the voluntary reporting of serious adverse events or product quality problems associated with medications through the _____ _____ form.

27. For patients to benefit from drug therapy, they must understand the importance of taking the medicine in the proper _____, at the recommended time, and in the _____ way.

28. Increasing the number of medications an individual receives not only increases the risk of interactions and adverse side effects, but also increases the risk of _____.

29. The health care practitioner should never _____ medication at the bedside unless specifically ordered by the physician.

30. The health care practitioner should _____ open the unit-dose packet until the patient is prepared to take the medicine.

Multiple Choice

Circle the letter that best answers the question.

1. Before administering medications to a patient, the health care practitioner should explain that:

    A. The physician always orders this medication regardless of patient diagnosis.
    B. Many medications look like the drug the physician ordered.
    C. Medication dosage may have changed.
    D. Preparation of the medication is difficult.

2. The policy and procedure book found at the agency where the health care provider is administering drugs is a resource:

    A. Just like the *PDR* or the *AHFS Drug Information*.
    B. Outlining the rules and regulations for medication administration at that particular institution or agency.
    C. Explaining how the drugs were made and which medications are control substances.
    D. Describing which patients should receive which medications according to the medical diagnosis.

3. When administering medications, the health care practitioner should:

   A. Leave medications at the bedside for the patient to take when he or she wakes up.
   B. Give medication that someone else prepared.
   C. Confirm the right medication for the patient.
   D. Open all packets, even unit-dose packs, before entering the patient's room.

4. The health care practitioner is preparing a medication to a patient that requires conversion to another system. Before administering the medication the health care practitioner should:

   A. Estimate the correct answer.
   B. Check the calculations with another trained health care practitioner, pharmacist, or doctor.
   C. Substitute a liquid medication form for a tablet or capsule when a patient has difficulty swallowing.
   D. Always recheck the dose if only one tablets is to be given.

5. The route of administration of a medication is important because it effects which of these?

   A. Degree of absorption.
   B. Cost to the patient.
   C. Patient's cooperation in taking the medication.
   D. Ease of preparation by the health care practitioner.

6. If no route is specified in the physician's order, which route would be used by the health care practitioner unless conditions warrant otherwise?

   A. Oral
   B. Intramuscular
   C. Subcutaneous
   D. Intravenous

7. When it becomes necessary for the health care practitioner to destroy narcotics because of partial dosage, cancellation, or error, the documentation should include:

   A. Flushing all medications down the toilet and documenting that the patient did not receive the medication.
   B. Placing the medications in the stock drawer for another patient.
   C. Securing the narcotic in the patient's drawer or room for the next dosage.
   D. Having two health care practitioners sign as witnesses of the disposal of the drug.

8. What actions has the FDA taken in response to the voluntary reports on the MED WATCH forms from the health care community?

   A. Filed suit against the facility where the patient was receiving treatment.
   B. Set up opposition action toward the individual health care practitioners who filled out the reports.
   C. Issued warnings, made labeling changes, required manufacturers to do post-marketing studies, and ordered withdrawal of products from the market.
   D. Worked together with the facility involved to assist the patients who were affected by the products whether in a positive way or negative way.

9. While medication errors can and do occur in all health care settings, more errors are reported from which settings?

   A. Acute care
   B. Outpatient
   C. Long-term care
   D. Ambulatory care

10. When a mistake is made in the administration of medication(s), the health care practitioner should do which of the following first?

   A. Report it immediately to the one in charge so that corrective action can be taken.
   B. Apologize to the nursing staff, the physician, and the other health care practitioners.
   C. Complete a written incident report as a legal requirement.
   D. Ask the patient not to file a civil suit against the health care provider.

Matching A

Match the "right" of medication administration in Column A with the description in Column B.

COLUMN A	COLUMN B
_____ 1. Right medication	A. Checking the patient's identification band and asking the client to state his name
_____ 2. Right amount	B. Administering a medication that is prescribed once a day pc after the client eats breakfast
_____ 3. Right time	C. Carefully compares the dosage ordered with the dose on hand (the unit-dose packet)
_____ 4. Right route	D. Calling the physician to question giving a medication orally when the client's ability to swallow has decreased
_____ 5. Right patient	E. Cautiously compares the name or the drug prescribed with the label on the package, bottle, or unit-dose pack
_____ 6. Right documentation	F. Recording the time the pain medication was given, along with the dosage, route, and location if an injection

Matching B

Match the action of the health care provider administering medications in Column A with the responsibility in Column B.

COLUMN A	COLUMN B
_____ 1. Observing the patient's vital signs before administering a medication	A. Assessment
_____ 2. Writing the results of a medication on the patient's chart	B. Intervention
_____ 3. Taking steps to counteract an adverse reaction	C. Evaluation
_____ 4. Taking a complete history, including all medical conditions	D. Documentation
_____ 5. Asking the patient if the medication has relieved his pain	
_____ 6. Identifying any allergies the patient may have	
_____ 7. Appropriate judgment in timing and discontinuing a medication if required	
_____ 8. Responding to a severe hypersensitivity response	

True or False

Circle T for true or F for false after reading each of the following statements.

1. T F It is essential to scrutinize every letter in the name of the medication when comparing the medicine ordered with the medicine on hand.

2. T F It is the responsibility of the health care practitioner administering medications to have the wisdom and judgment to accurately assess the patient's needs for the medication ordered.

3. T F The health care provider administering medications should first administer the medication and then assess the patient's need for the medication.

4. T F One of the major responsibilities of the health care provider in drug administration is skill in accurate delivery of the medication, in the best interests of the patients.

5. T F The health care provider administering drugs is responsible to provide patient education about medications administered.

6. T F Administer medications on time even the medication is poured from a bottle without a clear label.

7. T F Insist that the patient take the medication even if he questions the size of the pill; it is probably a different manufacturer.

8. T F Before giving a medication ordered by the physician, confirm the patient's identity by checking name and identification number on the patient wristband.

9. T F The health care practitioner must label a medication if it is stored in an unlabeled container before it is considered the right medication to administer.

10. T F The health care provider administering medications must pay close attention to the patient's questions about his or her medications or the dosage of medication he or she is receiving.

11. T F An unusual dosage of a medication should alert the health care practitioner to the possibility of an error.

12. T F Some medications need to be maintained at a specific level in the blood and are therefore prescribed TID.

13. T F Many medications that are irritating to the stomach are ordered to be administered ac or before meals.

14. T F Patient education includes instruction about the right time to take specific medicines and why.

15. T F The route of administration may not be changed without a physician's order even though a change is indicated because of a client's condition.

16. T F When a patient's record is examined in court, the accuracy of medication documentation can be a critical factor in some legal judgments.

17. T F MEDWATCH encourages the health care practitioner to regard voluntary reporting of serious, adverse events or product quality problems associated with medications regulated by the FDA as a part of his or her professional responsibility.

18. T F The health care practitioner can administer medications that have been prepared by anyone on the health care team.

Administration by the Gastrointestinal Route

Fill-in-the-Blank

Fill in the blank for each of the following statements.

1. Gastrointestinal administration includes four categories: oral, nasogastric tube, _____ _____, and rectal.

2. A major advantage of administering medications via the nasogastric tube is the ability to bypass the _____ and _____ when necessary.

3. In some situations the surgeon may insert a gastric tube through the skin of the abdomen directly into the _____ after the patient has been unable to take _____ for extended periods of time.

4. Medications administered via the _____ route are able to bypass the actions of the digestive enzymes.

5. _____ of medications administered by the rectal route may be irregular or incomplete if feces are present.

6. After locating the medication in the medication cupboard or cart, the health care practitioner should compare the _____ against the medication record for the Five Rights of Medication Administration.

7. The first guideline, whether administering medications orally, via a nasogastric tube, or rectally is to complete a medical asepsis _____.

8. It is the health care practitioner's responsibility prior to administering medications to know the _____ of the drug, possible side effects, contraindications, cautions, interactions, and normal _____ range.

9. Prior to administering medications the health care practitioner should verify that the patient's identity by asking the patient to state his or her name and date of _____ and compare this information with that on the medication record.

10. The health care practitioner should always assess and record a patient's _____ _____ before administering an antihypertensive medication.

11. When a patient is NPO for surgery, has nausea or dysphagia, the doctor may need to be consulted regarding a change of _____ since medications should not be omitted completely without specific instructions.

12. The health care practitioner should administer oral medications with _____, unless otherwise ordered, and stay with the patient until the medication has been _____.

© 2011 Cengage Learning. All Rights Reserved. May not be scanned, copied or duplicated, or posted to a publicly accessible website, in whole or in part.

13. Medications whose action depends on contact with the mucous membranes of the mouth or throat should not be administered with any fluid or _____.

14. When preparing liquid medications, the health care practitioner should hold the medicine cup at eye _____ and place the _____ on the level to which the medicine will be poured.

15. When liquid medication needs to be administered via a syringe, the health care practitioner should first pour the prescribed medication into a _____ _____ and then withdraw the prescribed amount of medication in a syringe.

16. When administering a liquid medication via syringe, place the syringe tip in the pocket between the cheek and _____ and instill the medication slowly to lessen chances of aspiration.

17. One method of checking placement of a nasogastric tube prior to administration of medication via the NG tube is to _____ stomach contents with a syringe and verify that the contents have a pH of 0.9 to _____.

18. While administering medication via a nasogastric tube, the health care practitioner should always allow the medication to flow by _____ and never force fluids down the tube.

19. When the health care practitioner administers medications rectally, it is important to remember to respect the patient's _____ and privacy by closing the door and not exposing the patient unnecessarily.

20. When administering medications rectally or via a nasogastric tube to a patient who is unconscious, the health care practitioner should always _____ everything being done and why.

21. Rectal medications may be in the form of a _____ or administered as a retention enema.

22. After administering a retention enema, the health care practitioner should instruct the patient to lie quietly on either _____ to aid in retention of the medication.

23. When administering a suppository to an infant, the health care practitioner should use a gloved _____ finger.

24. Prior to administration of a suppository, the health care practitioner should position the patient on the _____ side with the knee in flexed position.

Multiple Choice

Circle the letter that best answers the question.

1. Which of the following best describes an advantage of administering medications by the oral route?

    A. Cannot be used when the patient is nauseated or vomiting
    B. Slower onset of absorption and action when trying to relieve pain
    C. Potential of aspiration for a patient with an altered level of consciousness or dysphagia
    D. Medication can be retrieved in case of error or intentional overdose

2. When a patient is unable to swallow for prolonged periods of time because of illness, trauma, surgery, or decreased level of consciousness, which route of medication is often ordered?

    A. Intravenous
    B. Oral
    C. Nasogastric tube
    D. Intramuscular injection

3. What term describes a tube can be secured in place indefinitely for feeding purposes and medication administration directly into the stomach through the abdominal wall?

    A. Nasogastric
    B. PEG
    C. Rectal
    D. Oral

4. When administering oral medications, the health care practitioner should never:

   A. Administer drugs with applesauce.
   B. Elevate the patient's head above 30 degrees.
   C. Give the cardiac medication before the vitamin.
   D. Open or crush timed-release capsules or enteric-coated tablets.

5. The health care practitioner knows that medications should not be administered via the GI route if they are:

   A. Discolored
   B. Scored tablets
   C. Refrigerated liquids
   D. Suspensions

6. If a patient vomits within 20 to 30 minutes after administration of an oral medication, the health care practitioner should:

   A. Report the occurrence to the person in charge.
   B. Repeat the medication.
   C. Ask the patient to take slow deep breaths.
   D. Observe for toxic effects of drugs.

7. When a patient refuses to take a medication by mouth or is NPO for some reason, the health care practitioner should:

   A. Change the route but not the medication.
   B. Ask the person in charge to change the route or medication.
   C. Change the order and have the physician sign it in the near future.
   D. Call the physician to request a written order for change of route.

8. If a patient on intermittent suction is receiving a medication via the nasogastric tube, the suction to the tube should be turned off for how long for the medication to be absorbed?

   A. 10 minutes
   B. 15 minutes
   C. 20 minutes
   D. 30 minutes

9. When administering a retention enema, the health care practitioner is aware that the solution must be retained approximately:

   A. 10 minutes.
   B. 15 minutes.
   C. 20 minutes.
   D. 30 minutes.

10. When administering a rectal suppository, the health care practitioner should:

    A. Leave the wrapper on and insert the suppository approximately 2 inches above the internal sphincter.
    B. Remove the wrapper and lubricate the widest end and insert approximately 1 inch above the internal sphincter.
    C. Administer the suppository with a gloved hand after lubricating the tapered end by inserting it just past the internal sphincter.
    D. Insert the suppository the length of the little finger after placing the patient in a sitting position and lubricating the suppository.

Matching

Match the order of the steps for administration of medications via a nasogastric tube in Column A with the order number of the step in Column B.

	COLUMN A	COLUMN B
_____ 1.	Hold the end of the tube up and remove the clamp, plug, or adapter.	A. 1st
_____ 2.	Check the identification bracelet, ask the patient his or her name, and elevate the head of the bed if not contraindicated.	B. 2nd
_____ 3.	Place a stethoscope over the patient's stomach, attach the syringe to the tube, and inject about 30 mL of air, listening for a swooshing sound as the air enters the stomach.	C. 3rd
_____ 4.	Leave the syringe attached firmly to the tubing and remove the plunger or bulb from the syringe after clamping the tube with your fingers (bend it over itself or pinch it).	D. 4th
_____ 5.	Document the correct placement of the nasogastric tube and the administration of the medication via the tube.	E. 5th
_____ 6.	Begin flushing the tube by adding 60–100 mL of water to the syringe just before the syringe has emptied of the medication.	F. 6th
_____ 7.	Position the patient on his or her right side and/or elevate the head of the bed to encourage the stomach to empty while also maintaining comfort.	G. 7th
_____ 8.	Check the medication order using the five rights of medication administration.	H. 8th
_____ 9.	Release or unclamp the tube after you have begun to pour the medication into the syringe (medication should flow by gravity).	I. 9th
_____ 10.	Wash hands and put on gloves.	J. 10th
_____ 11.	After the water flushing the tube has run in, pinch the tube, remove the syringe, and clamp or plug the tube.	K. 11th
_____ 12.	Prepare the medication as ordered and take it to the patient's room, being sure the medication is at room temperature.	L. 12th

True or False

Circle T for true or F for false after reading each of the following statements.

1. T F A major advantage of using the nasogastric tube for administration of medications is that there is very little discomfort even for the alert patient.

2. T F Medications available in suppository form can be administered to the patient suffering from dysphagia.

3. T F If a patient expresses any doubts about a medication being administered, the health care practitioner should recheck the medication order.

4. T F The only time the health care practitioner is required to document about medication administration is when there is an adverse reaction.

5. T F When a patient is NPO, prescribed medications are omitted and resumed on the following day.

6. T F When administering a medication orally or nasogastric tube, the health care practitioner should elevate the patient's head, if not contraindicated by the patient's condition, to assist in swallowing.

7. T F Tablets that must be divided should be broken by hand so that the patient can take one half of the tablet.

8. T F When administering more than one medication, the health care practitioner should give the most important medication first.

9. T F When the patient vomits after taking medications orally, the health care practitioner should document on the patient's record the time of emesis and its appearance.

10. T F When preparing liquid medications, the health care practitioner should hold the medicine bottle with the label side upward to prevent smearing of the label while pouring.

11. T F The health care practitioner should keep the head of the bed flat when administering liquid medications via a syringe to avoid aspiration.

12. T F When administering large amounts of liquid medication via syringe, place a 2-inch length of latex tubing on the syringe tip to facilitate instillation into the cheek pocket.

13. T F A nasogastric tube is often inserted solely for the administration of medications.

14. T F When checking for proper placement of the nasogastric tube, the health care practitioner listens with a stethoscope for a whooshing sound over the patient's stomach while injecting 30 mL of air into the NG tube.

15. T F When checking the gastric aspirate for proper placement of the nasogastric tube, the health care practitioner knows the gastric juice has a pH of 2–3.

16. T F When administering medications by gastric tube checking for placement of the tube is optional.

17. T F After the health care practitioner administers a retention enema, the patient should be allowed to go directly to the bathroom and expel the contents.

18. T F The health care practitioner administering a suppository should ask the patient to take a deep breath just prior to inserting the suppository gently into the rectum.

CHAPTER 9

Administration by the Parenteral Route

Fill-in-the-Blank

Fill in the blank for each of the following statements.

1. Administration of medications via the sublingual, buccal, transcutaneous inhalation and injection parenteral routes produce _____ effects.

2. Transcutaneous or _____ systems deliver the medication to the body by absorption through the skin.

3. After applying the transdermal patch, the health care practitioner should write the date and _____ on the patch.

4. To reduce the occurrence of headaches, physicians may order nitroglycerin ointment or a Transdermal-Nitro patch to be applied at _____ and removed the next day at noon.

5. Potent drugs may be given via inhalation therapy in small amounts, _____ the side effects.

6. Effective inhalation therapy requires cooperation of the patient in proper _____ techniques and the ability to follow directions for the medication administration.

7. One disadvantage of inhalation therapy is that patients who have asthma or chronic obstructive pulmonary disease (COPD) sometimes become _____ on a small-volume nebulizer or MDI.

8. For effective medication administration via the metered dose inhaler (MDI), the patient must understand and follow correct _____ techniques.

9. A _____ may be added to the metered dose inhaler to act as a reservoir for the aerosol, allowing the patient to first depress the canister and then inhale.

10. The health care practitioner should teach the patient to hold his/her breath for _____ to _____ seconds after inhaling the medication slowly and deeply.

11. Proper daily _____ of small-volume nebulizers is essential to avoid infection.

12. The health care practitioner should instruct the patient receiving medication using the small-volume nebulizer not to take any other _____, including over-the-counter drugs, without the doctor's permission in order to avoid serious side effects.

13. Intermittent positive-pressure breathing treatments combines administration of an aerosol with a mechanical _____ to assist patients who are unable to take a deep breath on their own.

14. The _____ of the syringe is the outer, hollow cylinder that holds the medication and has calibrations for measuring the quantity of medication to be given.

15. The health care practitioner preparing to administer an injection is aware that the length of the needle depends on the _____ of injection and the size of the patient.

16. The _____ of the needle refers to the size of the lumen or the diameter of the shaft and is numbered in reverse order.

17. The thinner needle with the _____ diameter has the larger gauge number.

18. All insulin dosages should be _____-_____ by two health caregivers before administration.

19. Each calibration for a U-100 insulin _____ has a dual scale: even numbers on one side and odd numbers on the other side.

20. Lo-Dose _____ syringes have calibrations of only one unit, making it extremely important for the health care practitioner to study the calibrations carefully each time an insulin injection is prepared.

21. A _____ syringe is a premeasured amount of medication contained in the syringe.

22. The health care practitioner is aware that only _____ needles are to be recapped.

23. When opening an ampule to draw up medication, the health care practitioner should hold the tip of the ampule with an alcohol wipe and break the ampule open along the scored _____ at the neck.

24. When two drugs are to be combined in a syringe, the health care practitioner must first check for _____ of drugs to be administered.

25. After the health care practitioner has administered an intradermal injection, the patient will have a visible bubble or _____ at the site of the injection.

26. The Z-track method is used for injections that are irritating to the tissue, such as iron _____, hydroxyzine or cephazolin.

27. With all intramuscular injections the health care practitioner will _____ by pulling back on the plunger and _____ the needle if any blood appears in the syringe.

28. If eyedrops and ointment are ordered for the same time, instill _____ first, wait 5 minutes, then apply the _____.

29. After positioning the patient with the head back, the health care practitioner uses aseptic technique to instill the correct number of eyedrops or ointment dosage into the lower _____ sac.

30. The health care practitioner should apply gentle pressure on the inner _____ following administration of ophthalmic medications to minimize systemic absorption with medications such as corticosteroids, miotics, and mydriatics.

Multiple Choice

Circle the letter that best answers the question.

1. Which of the following medications affect the body as a whole with systemic effects rather than local effects?

    A. Eye ointment
    B. Eardrops
    C. Triple antibiotic ointment
    D. Transdermal patch

2. A medication administered under the tongue uses what route?

    A. Sublingual
    B. Transcutaneous
    C. Intradermal
    D. Buccal

3. When the health care practitioner provides patient education for medications administered by the sublingual or buccal route, which of the following instructions should be included?

    A. Do not drink or take food until the medication is completely absorbed.
    B. Swallow the medication after holding it in place for approximately 30 seconds.
    C. Breathe in as the medication is inhaled during inspiration.
    D. Massage the medication into the skin and apply a cover over the site.

4. Which of the following medications would be placed behind the ear and left in place for up to 72 hours, as necessary, to prevent motion sickness?

   A. Durgesic patch
   B. Nitroglycerin ointment
   C. Transderm-Nitro
   D. Scopolamine patch

5. When teaching a patient to administer nitroglycerin ointment, which of these steps should be done **first**?

   A. Avoid touching the ointment without gloves on.
   B. Rotate sites for application.
   C. Apply the prescribed amount of ointment onto Appli-Ruler paper.
   D. Shave the application area.

6. One metered dose inhaler (MDI) completely full will provide approximately how many puffs of medication?

   A. 50
   B. 100
   C. 150
   D. 200

7. The health care practitioner is teaching a patient to administer an inhaled steroid medication and a bronchodilator that are to be given at the same time. What is the correct administration technique?

   A. Wash the mouth out with tap water, inhale the bronchodilator, wait 10 minutes and inhale the steroid.
   B. Inhale the steroid, wait 15 minutes, and administer two puffs of the bronchodilator.
   C. Administer the bronchodilator first, then after 1 to 2 minutes administer the steroid followed by rinsing the mouth with tap water.
   D. Administer the steroid, rinse the mouth, and immediately administer the bronchodilator.

8. A patient has been instructed in how to properly clean a small-volume nebulizer. The health care practitioner recognizes more teaching is required if the patient states which of the following?

   A. First, disassemble the pieces of the nebulizer, wash in mild soapy water, and rinse thoroughly.
   B. Second, soak the pieces of the nebulizer in a solution of two parts vinegar and one part water for 20–30 minutes.
   C. After removing the nebulizer parts from the vinegar solution, rinse with warm tap water.
   D. After the nebulizer parts are completely dry reassemble for next use.

9. When administering an intermittent positive-pressure breathing treatment, the health care practitioner should:

   A. Monitor vital signs closely, watching for a tachycardia and decreased or shallow respirations.
   B. Check for a sudden rise in blood pressure.
   C. Ask the patient to cough after each inhalation.
   D. Save all sputum expelled.

10. The inner, solid rod that fits snugly into the cylinder that allows the health care practitioner to draw medication into the syringe or eject solution or air from the syringe is called a:

    A. Shaft.
    B. Hub.
    C. Bevel.
    D. Plunger.

11. Which of the following best describes the shaft of the needle?

    A. The long hollow tubes varying in lengths and gauges, embedded in the hub
    B. The inner solid rod that fits snugly into the cylinder
    C. The pointed end with a beveled edge
    D. The portion that holds the needle with a Luer-Lok

12. Which of the following parts of a syringe must remain sterile during the preparation and administration of an injectable medication?

    A. The plunger only
    B. The needle and plunger
    C. Inside and the tip of the barrel and the needle
    D. Inside and the tip of the barrel, the plunger, and the needle

13. When correctly drawing up a medication from a vial, the health care practitioner would first:

    A. Insert the needle into the center of the rubber diaphragm and withdraw the correct amount of medication.
    B. Invert the vial, insert the needle, and withdraw the prescribed dosage of medication.
    C. Draw air into the syringe equal to the amount of medication to be withdrawn from the vial.
    D. Remove all air bubbles from the solution and withdraw the needle from the vial.

14. Which of these terms describes the special needle required by some health care facilities to withdraw fluid from an ampule?

    A. Cartridge
    B. Filter
    C. Carpuject
    D. Standard

15. Which of the following describes the correct technique for administering an intradermal injection?

    A. Pinch the skin into a fat fold of at least 1 inch, insert the 5/8-inch needle at a 45-degree angle, and inject the medication slowly.
    B. Stretch the skin taut at the injection site, insert a 1-inch needle at a 90-degree angle, withdraw the needle rapidly, holding a 2 × 2 gauze over the site.
    C. Stretch the skin as far as you can to the outer side and hold it there, insert the 1-inch needle at a 90-degree angle; after removing the needle, allow the skin to return to normal position.
    D. Stretch the skin taut, insert the 3/8-inch needle with bevel up at a 10–15 degree angle, and inject slowly, forming a bubble just under the skin.

16. The health care practitioner should adhere to which of the following techniques for intradermal injections?

    A. Inject the medication very slowly, observing for a small white bubble.
    B. If no bubble forms, withdraw the needle and use another site.
    C. Aspirate before injecting the medication.
    D. Massage injection site; apply gentle pressure with a dry 2 × 2 gauze.

17. Patient instructions after administration of an intradermal injection should include which of these verbal and written instructions?

    A. Keep the area covered with a Band-Aid.
    B. Avoid scrubbing, scratching, or rubbing the area of the injection.
    C. Return to the health care facility the following week for follow-up.
    D. Clean the area every 4 hours with soap and water for at least 48 hours.

18. The Z-track method is used for IM injections of iron preparations. Which intramuscular site is the site for this type of injection?

    A. Rectus femoris
    B. Deltoid
    C. Ventrogluteal
    D. Dorsogluteal

19. What should the health care practitioner do after aspirating and seeing blood in the syringe when administering an intramuscular injection?

    A. Remove and discard the syringe with the needle uncapped.
    B. Remove the needle and syringe and recap.
    C. Continue with the injection because this is a normal finding.
    D. Inject the medication slowly in case it is in a vessel.

20. When more than one eye medication is ordered, how much time should the health care practitioner wait before instilling the second medication?

   A. 2 minutes
   B. 3 minutes
   C. 4 minutes
   D. 5 minutes

Matching A

Match the type of injection and/or the patient receiving the injection in Column A with the syringe type, length, and needle gauge in Column B.

COLUMN A	COLUMN B
____ 1. Subcutaneous insulin	A. Tuberculin, 5/8 inch, 25 gauge
____ 2. Intramuscular, Z-track	B. Insulin U-100, 3/8 inch, 26 gauge
____ 3. Intradermal	C. 3 mL, 2-inch, 21 gauge
____ 4. Intramuscular, children and thin adults	D. Tuberculin, 3/8 inch, 27 gauge
____ 5. Intramuscular, larger adult	E. 3 mL, 1-inch, 22 gauge
____ 6. Subcutaneous heparin	F. 3 mL, 2-inch, 19 gauge

Matching B

Match the description of the preferred patient or the location of injection site for intramuscular injections in Column A with the injection site in Column B. Note that the injection sites in Column B can be used more than once.

COLUMN A	COLUMN B
____ 1. Preferred site for infants	A. Dorsogluteal
____ 2. Upper outer arm above the axilla and below the acromium	B. Ventrogluteal
____ 3. Not used for children under 3 years old	C. Deltoid
____ 4. Front of the thigh toward the outside of the leg	D. Vastus lateralis
____ 5. Front of the thigh toward the midline of the leg	E. Rectus femoris
____ 6. Can be used for all patients	
____ 7. Not good for older adults, nonambulatory, or emaciated patients	
____ 8. Only used for patients requiring 1 mL or less	
____ 9. One handbreadth above the knee and one handbreadth below the greater trochanter toward the outside of the leg	
____ 10. One handbreadth above the knee and one handbreadth below the greater trochanter toward the midline of the leg	
____ 11. Inject in a V, formed by placing the palm on the greater trochanter, the index finger on the anterior superior iliac spine, and the middle finger on the iliac crest	
____ 12. Upper outer quadrant of the buttock	

True or False

Circle T for true or F for false after reading each of the following statements.

1. T F Local effects are those limited to one particular part (location) of the body, with very little, if any, effect on the rest of the body.

2. T F One major advantage of medications administered by the sublingual route is that medications absorbed in this way are unaffected by the stomach, intestines, or liver.

3. T F With administration of medications via the buccal route the health care practitioner would place the medication under the tongue.

4. T F Nitroglycerin ointment is administered intradermally in prescribed amounts every few hours for prevention of angina pectoris.

5. T F Absorption of medications administered by the transcutaneous delivery system is slower, but the action is more prolonged than with other methods of administration.

6. T F Estraderm is a transdermal form of estrogen ordered by some physicians.

7. T F One of the advantages of inhalation therapy is the rapid action of the drug, with local effects within the respiratory tract.

8. T F When inhalation therapy is administered infrequently, the patient will likely experience irritation of the trachea or bronchi or bronchospasm.

9. T F When using the metered dose inhaler (MDI), older adult patients may have difficulty coordinating the depression of the canister and inhaling at the same time.

10. T F Metered dose inhalers (MDIs) may be used in pediatrics with a mouthpiece or mask.

11. T F All patients receiving medication using the small-volume nebulizer should be cautioned by the health care practitioner to rise slowly from a reclining position to help prevent dizziness.

12. T F The tip of the syringe is the hollow cylinder that holds the medication.

13. T F The tuberculin syringe is used for injections requiring less than 1 mL of substance and is calibrated in tenths of a milliliter and in minims.

14. T F The Carpuject is an example of a disposable cartridge with a premeasured amount of medication that can be attached to a holder and used to access a needleless IV system or with an attached needle to administer an intramuscular or subcutaneous injection.

15. T F When drawing up medication from a vial that has been previously opened, the health care practitioner will wipe the rubber diaphragm with one part vinegar and two parts water.

16. T F The health care practitioner is aware that sterile needles may be recapped, maintaining sterility and preventing needle sticks.

17. T F The health care practitioner administering a subcutaneous heparin injection should not aspirate prior to injecting the medication slowly or massage the injection area after removing the needle.

18. T F After aspirating the IM injection, the health care practitioner is aware that if blood is seen in the syringe the needle should be withdrawn and injected into another IM site.

19. T F The health care practitioner administering an intramuscular injection will insert the needle at a 90 degree angle with a quick, dartlike motion of the dominant hand.

20. T F Advise the patient after receiving a Z-track IM injection that walking will aid absorption and that she should avoid tight garments, such as girdles, that cause pressure on the site.

CHAPTER 10

Poison Control

Fill-in-the-Blank

Fill in the blank for each of the following statements.

1. Poisonings are the leading cause of health emergencies for _____ in the nation.

2. Children between the ages of one and _____5_____ are at greatest risk for poisoning.

3. In 2004, the American Academy of Pediatrics (AAP) changed its policy statement in relation to poison treatment in the home by recommending against keeping _____ in the home and that any of this medication presently in homes be disposed of safely.

4. The first step to take in any suspected poisoning is to contact the local _____ _____ _____.

5. The _____ _____ _____ can give instructions by phone for appropriate emergency treatment after the caller gives the details on the type of poison and the patient's condition, age, and weight.

6. To induce vomiting in a patient who has ingested gasoline, kerosene, or lighter fluid can cause aspiration and/or _oxfixiation_.

7. Gastric lavage is not used in patients who have ingested _kerosene_ substances because of the danger of perforating the damaged tissue of the esophagus.

8. When a patient is poisoned with a central nervous system (CNS) depressant, an _medication_ such as a CNS stimulant may be required.

9. The patient being treated for poisoning by inhalation requires symptomatic treatment, including fresh air, CPR, and _____ if indicated.

10. Poisoning by an insect sting should be treated by cleansing the area, applying _____, and immediately removing the stinger of a bee or wasp.

11. The health care practitioner should always observe the patient with an allergy to an insect sting for possible _____ reaction.

12. The health care practitioner can play a major role in reducing the number of _____ poisonings in children by stressing preventive measures to parents.

Note: Numbers 13–26 are precautions recommended by the American Medical Association to prevent poisoning.

13. Keep all medications, household chemicals, cleaning supplies, and pesticides in a _____ cupboard.

14. Never store poisonous _____ in the same area with food as confusion could be fatal.

15. Never reuse containers of _____ products.

16. When discarding medications, consult your _pharmacy_ about proper disposal in your area.

17. Do not give or take medications in the _dark_.

18. Never leave _Medication_ on a bedside stand.

19. Always _____ the label before taking medication or pouring any solution for ingestion.

20. Never tell children the medication you are giving them is _candy_.

21. When preparing a baby's formula, _taste_ the ingredients.

22. Never give or _____ any medications that are discolored, have a strange odor, or are outdated.

23. Don't take medication in front of _____.

24. Keep pocketbooks, purses, and pillboxes out of the _____ of children.

25. Rinse out containers thoroughly before _____ of them.

26. The National Poison Control Center toll-free number is 1-800-222-_1222_.

27. Some patients who are allergic to insect stings carry a kit with medication prescribed by their _data_ for self-injection or injection by someone else.

28. There are more than seventy poison control centers throughout the United States and Canada with computerized _Data_ to give you the latest information about poisons.

29. The health care practitioner should instruct patients to obtain the telephone number of their nearest poison control center and place it near or on their _telephone_.

Multiple Choice

Circle the letter that best answers the question.

1. Which of the following may occur in patients with cardiac or vascular disease if vomiting is induced as a treatment for poisoning?

    A. Decrease blood pressure and heart block
    B. Stroke and cardiac arrhythmias
    C. Urinary retention and low blood pressure
    D. Decreased heart rate and sinus arrhythmias

2. For a patient who has taken any kind of poison, the health care practitioner should prepare to:

    A. Administer gastric lavage and save any emesis.
    B. Administer activated charcoal before and after inducing emesis.
    C. Observe the patient closely for confusion, tremors, and convulsions.
    D. Notify the nearest Poison Control Center.

3. For a patient who has experienced external poisoning of the skin or eyes, the health care practitioner should flush the affected area with a continuous stream of water for at least how many minutes?

    A. 2 to 5
    B. 6 to 10
    C. 11 to 15
    D. 20 to 30

4. Appropriate treatment for a patient with snakebite includes:

    A. Applying a tourniquet above the site.
    B. Putting an ice pack directly on the site.
    C. Keeping the patient quiet in order to slow circulation.
    D. Transporting the patient in an upright position to an emergency care facility.

5. After emergency care for a insect sting, the health care practitioner should instruct the patient to apply which of these ointments to the area?

   A. Silvadene
   B. Lidocaine
   C. Testosterone
   D. Corticosteroid

6. The Food and Drug Administration (FDA) reports that iron pills are the leading cause of poisoning deaths in children under what age?

   A. 6 months
   B. 6 years
   C. 10 months
   D. 10 years

7. The health care practitioner is aware that older adults are at risk for poisoning because of toxic reactions that possibly result from:

   A. Taking the wrong dosage due to impaired vision or poor memory.
   B. Having a more rapid metabolism.
   C. Having family members dispense the patient's medications.
   D. Increased absorption of most medications.

8. A patient experiencing systemic absorption of poisons through the skin may require administration of which of these?

   A. An antidote
   B. A topical corticosteroid
   C. Oxygen and fresh air
   D. An antivenom

9. Carbon monoxide poisoning can quickly rob the tissues of what vital substance?

   A. Oxygen
   B. Carbon dioxide
   C. Nitrogen
   D. Hemoglobin

Matching

Match the definition in Column A with the term in Column B.

COLUMN A	COLUMN B
_____ 1. Pertaining to a matter or substance that causes vomiting	A. Activated charcoal
_____ 2. Minimizes systemic absorption of ingested poison	B. Corrosive
_____ 3. The oral taking of substance into the body	C. Antivenom (antivenin)
_____ 4. Any matter or substance that interferes with normal physiological function when inhaled, ingested, injected, or absorbed in the body	D. Antidote
_____ 5. A drug or other substance that counters the action of a poison	E. Emetic
_____ 6. Eating away a tissue or substance, especially by chemical action	F. Ingestion
_____ 7. The rinsing or washing out of the stomach with a saline solution or sterile water	G. Gastric lavage
_____ 8. A suspension prepared from the serum of immunized horses of venom-neutralizing antibodies	H. Poison

True or False

Circle T for true or F for false after reading each of the following statements.

1. T F The health care practitioner is aware that, with ingestion of corrosive substances such as ammonia or dishwasher detergent, vomiting should be induced as soon as possible.

2. T F Inducing vomiting in the patient who is semiconscious, severely inebriated, in shock, or convulsing could cause choking, aspiration, and/or asphyxiation.

3. T F If perforation of the patient's esophagus occurs as a result of poisoning, surgery will be required.

4. T F Sometimes a substance such as activated charcoal is administered after emesis or gastric lavage to minimize systemic absorption of an ingested poison.

5. T F Cardiopulmonary resuscitation (CPR) may be required for the patient who is poisoned by a CNS depressant.

6. T F The health care practitioner should instruct the patient to apply ice or a tourniquet after a snakebite.

7. T F The physician may order urine and blood tests for toxicology if there is doubt about the type of poison or the amount absorbed.

8. T F When a patient suffers from a snakebite, the caregiver should be instructed to transport the patient lying down to an emergency care facility for antivenom injections.

9. T F Vomiting is the first intervention with a patient who has ingested gasoline, lighter fluid, or kerosene.

10. T F Vomiting should never be induced in a child less than one year of age no matter what the poison.

11. T F Gastric lavage is not used in patients who have ingested corrosives because of the danger of perforating the damaged tissue of the esophagus.

12. T F Inhaling insect spray may require administration of an antidote.

Drug Classifications

CHAPTER 11

Vitamins, Minerals, and Herbs

Fill-in-the-Blank

Fill in the blank for each of the following statements.

1. Health care practitioners should advise patients to _____ self-medication with large doses of vitamins or minerals, which may not be indicated if the diet is well balanced and the individual is in good health.

2. A need or _____ of vitamins or minerals should be established by a physician's diagnosis or blood test before exceeding the Recommended Dietary Allowances (RDA).

3. A major revision is currently under way to replace the Recommended Dietary Allowances (RDA) called the Dietary Reference _____ (DRI).

4. Research reports have indicated the possibility of damage to tissues with the intake of large quantities of vitamins, above the _____ , especially those stored in the fat cells of the body.

5. Vitamin A is a _____ soluble vitamin and is necessary for the resistance to infection, proper visual function at night, and maintaining healthy epithelial tissue.

6. Vitamin D is synthesized in the body through the action of _____ on the skin.

7. The difference between the therapeutic dosage of vitamin D and that causing hypercalcemia is very small, and dosage must be carefully _____ and regulated.

8. Vitamin E supplements should be discontinued 10 days prior to surgery because of the danger of _____ bleeding time.

9. Vitamin K is not effective for bleeding from causes such as _____ overdose.

10. Vitamin B_1 (thiamine) is a coenzyme utilized for _____ metabolism.

11. The health care practitioner instructs patients that vitamin B_1 is found in whole grains, wheat germ, peas and _____ , especially _____ and organ meats.

12. Vitamin B_2 (riboflavin) is a coenzyme utilized in the metabolism of glucose, fats, and _____ _____ .

13. The health care practitioner instructs patients that vitamin B_2 is found in milk, eggs, nuts, meats yeast, enriched bread, and _____ leafy vegetables.

14. The health care practitioner should instruct patients taking levodopa alone (not combined with carbidopa) not to take a vitamin B_6 supplement because it _____ the action of levodopa.

15. The absorption of Vitamin B_{12} (cyanocobalamin) depends on an _____ factor normally present in the gastric juice of humans.

16. The National Academy of Sciences now suggests that all Americans over the age of _____ begin taking a low-dose vitamin B_{12} supplement or regularly eat breakfast cereals that are fortified with the vitamin.

17. A deficiency of folic acid during pregnancy can result in neural tube defects, such as _____ _____ , in the newborn.

18. The health care practitioner should caution patients about taking folic acid without checking with the physician first because it may mask the diagnosis of _____ _____ .

19. Folic acid doses over the RDA could interfere with the action of oral contraceptives, barbiturates, _____ .

20. Niacin, a vitamin found in meat, chicken, fish, milk, eggs, green vegetables, cooked dry beans and peas, soybeans, nuts, peanut butter, and enriched cereal products, is included in the B-complex group and up to _____ mg can safely be consumed daily.

21. Vitamin C, found in fresh fruits and vegetables, is required for iron absorption, formation of intracellular substances, normal teeth, gums, and bones, and promoting _____ of wounds and bone fractures.

22. The correct ratio of fluids to electrolytes has to be balanced for _____ body functioning.

23. Sodium and chloride are the principal minerals in the _____ body fluids.

24. Excessive potassium in the blood or _____ is most often the result of severe impairment.

25. Calcium is a mineral component of bones and teeth and is absorbed in the small intestine with the help of vitamin _____ .

26. The RDA for calcium is 1,000–1,200 mg/day for everyone except for _____ women not receiving estrogen therapy.

27. When injected by an IV, calcium salts should be administered very slowly to prevent tissue necrosis or cardiac _____ .

28. Sources of iron include meat, egg yolks, _____ , and enriched cereals.

29. Zinc supplements should be administered with meals to minimize _____ _____ .

30. The Dietary Supplement Health and Education Act (DSHEA) of 1994 recognized supplements as distinct from food additives and drugs; thus food supplements are not subject to the same FDA scrutiny and _____ as food additives and drugs.

31. Research on antioxidants is ongoing; however, statistical findings at this time indicate that natural antioxidants in food are much more effective than _____ products.

Multiple Choice

Circle the letter that best answers the question.

1. The Recommended Dietary Allowances (RDA) for average, normal, healthy adults include daily:

   A. Food intake.
   B. Vitamin supplementation.
   C. Mineral supplementation.
   D. Food intake and supplements.

2. The health care practitioner should instruct patients that megadoses of vitamin or mineral supplementation should be taken:

   A. No more than once a week.
   B. Only after meals.
   C. Only when ordered by a physician.
   D. Early in the morning before eating breakfast.

3. Signs of deficiency of vitamin A include:

   A. Muscle spasms, poor tooth and bone structure, skeletal deformities
   B. Increased clotting time, hematuria, melena
   C. Mental depression, memory loss, tingling in the extremities
   D. Night blindness, dry eyes and skin, weight loss

4. Which of the following correctly describes the RDA and DRI recommendations for daily intake of vitamin A?

   A. 800–1,000 U; 700–3,300 mcg
   B. 400 U; 5–15 mcg
   C. 30 IU; 15–1,000 mg
   D. 60–80 mg; 90–120 mcg

5. What synthetic vitamin A product is sometimes prescribed for severe acne?

   A. Beta carotene.
   B. Isotretinoin.
   C. Tocopherol.
   D. Retinal.

6. The term hypervitaminosis A refers to:

   A. Toxic effects of overdose of vitamin A.
   B. A placebo effect related to insufficient intake of vitamin A.
   C. Long-term use of the recommended dosage of a vitamin A supplement.
   D. Chronic deficiency of vitamin A intake.

7. What are the current RDA and DRI recommendations for daily intake of vitamin D?

   A. 800–1,000 U; 700–3,000 mcg
   B. 400 U; 5–15 mcg
   C. 30 UI; 15–1,000 mg
   D. 60–80 mg; 90–120 mcg

8. Which of the following best describes the signs of deficiency of vitamin D?

   A. Muscle spasms, poor tooth and bone structure, skeletal deformities
   B. Increased clotting time, hematuria, melena
   C. Mental depression, memory loss, tingling in the extremities
   D. Night blindness, dry eyes and skin, weight loss

9. Vitamin E supplements should not be taken while on anticoagulant therapy because of increased risk of:

   A. Kidney disease.
   B. Blood clots.
   C. Bleeding.
   D. Stunted growth.

10. Which of the following correctly describes the RDA and DRI recommendations for daily intake of vitamin E?

    A. 800–1,000 U; 700–3,000 mcg
    B. 400 U; 5–15 mcg
    C. 30 UI; 15–1,000 mg
    D. 60–80 mg; 90–120 mcg

11. Which of the following statements about vitamin K is correct?

    A. Required for administration to infants at birth in some states to prevent hemorrhagic disease of the newborn.
    B. The preferred route of administration is intramuscularly.
    C. It is absorbed in the stomach.
    D. Best dietary sources are breads, fruits, and milk.

12. Which of the following correctly describes the RDA and DRI recommendations for daily intake of vitamin K?

    A. 800–1,000 U; 700–3,000 mcg
    B. 60–80 mg; 90–120 mcg
    C. 400 U; 5–15 mcg
    D. 30 IU; 15–1,000 mg

13. Signs of deficiency of vitamin K include

    A. Muscle spasms, poor tooth and bone structure, skeletal deformities
    B. Increased clotting time, hematuria, melena
    C. Mental depression, memory loss, tingling in the extremities
    D. Night blindness, dry eyes and skin, weight loss

14. Signs of vitamin B_2 deficiency include

    A. Anorexia and constipation, GI upset
    B. Cardiovascular problems
    C. Numbness of the hands and feet
    D. Inflammation of the tongue and cracking at the corners of the mouth

15. The health care practitioner is aware that a deficient intake of vitamin C may result in:

    A. Intestinal obstruction.
    B. Scurvy.
    C. Pellagra.
    D. Rickets.

16. The potential side effects of the intake of large quantities of vitamin C include:

    A. Gastric irritation, increased uric acid, and kidney stones.
    B. Postural hypotension and jaundice.
    C. Muscle or bone pain.
    D. Prolonged clotting times, petechiae, and bruising.

17. Electrolytes carry positive or negative electrical charges required for body activities, such as:

    A. Conduction of nerve impulses and beating of the heart.
    B. Smooth muscle contraction.
    C. Storage of nutrients in the liver.
    D. Protein catabolism.

18. The health care practitioner should instruct the patient who is taking an oral iron preparation to take the prescribed dose with:

    A. an antacid.
    B. coffee.
    C. milk.
    D. orange juice.

19. Lean meat, organ meats, oysters, poultry, fish, and whole grain breads and cereals are all rich sources of which one of the following minerals?

    A. Calcium
    B. Zinc
    C. Potassium
    D. Chloride

20. Signs of iron deficiency include

    A. Imbalance in gastric acidity and reduced taste perception
    B. Hypertension, osteomalacia, and presence of a goiter
    C. Vertigo, weakness, pallor, and irregular heartbeat
    D. Osteoporosis, increased clotting time, and muscle pathology

21. Under the Dietary Supplement Health and Education Act (DSHEA), once a dietary supplement is marketed, the FDA has the responsibility for showing that a dietary supplement is:

    A. Unsafe before it can take action to restrict the product's use.
    B. To be used cautiously by consumers.
    C. Appropriate for the uses its label claims.
    D. Safe for ingestion by the consumer.

22. Which of the following herbs can be taken for PMS and/or menopausal symptoms?

    A. Garlic and saw palmetto
    B. Soy, black cohosh, and licorice
    C. Ginger, feverfew, and echinacea
    D. Chamomile, melatonin, and valerian

23. When a consumer asks a health care practitioner about taking over the counter supplements, which of these answers would be most appropriate?

    A. Use of the term "natural" guarantees that a product is safe.
    B. Ingredients in products with the USP notation indicates that the manufacturer followed standards established by the U.S. Pharmacopoeia.
    C. Products made in the United States are considered safe.
    D. Compare prices and purchase those products that cost less.

24. Which of the following herbs are taken for insomnia?

    A. Licorice and saw palmetto
    B. Soy and glucosamine
    C. Capsaicin, feverfew, and echinacea
    D. Chamomile, melatonin, and valerian

Matching A

Match the vitamin in Column A with the name in Column B.

COLUMN A	COLUMN B
_____ 1. Vitamin A	A. Riboflavin
_____ 2. Vitamin B_1	B. Ascorbic acid
_____ 3. Vitamin B_2	C. Beta carotene
_____ 4. Vitamin B_6	D. Thiamine
_____ 5. Vitamin B_{12}	E. Phytonadione
_____ 6. Folic acid	F. Folate
_____ 7. Niacin	G. Calciferol
_____ 8. Vitamin C	H. Tocopherol
_____ 9. Vitamin D	I. Pyridoxine
_____ 10. Vitamin E	J. Cyanocobalamin
_____ 11. Vitamin K	K. Nicotinic acid

Matching B

Match the vitamin in Column A with the description in Column B. Note that the descriptions in Column B can be used more than once.

COLUMN A	COLUMN B
_____ 1. Vitamin A	A. Water soluble
_____ 2. Vitamin B_1	B. Fat soluble
_____ 3. Vitamin B_2	
_____ 4. Vitamin B_6	

(*Matching continued on next page*)

COLUMN A
(continued)

_____ 5. Vitamin B_{12}

_____ 6. Folic acid

_____ 7. Niacin

_____ 8. Vitamin C

_____ 9. Vitamin D

_____ 10. Vitamin E

_____ 11. Vitamin K

True or False

Circle T for true or F for false after reading each of the following statements.

1. T F During pregnancy and lactation, vitamin and mineral supplementation are indicated, especially iron and calcium.

2. T F Chronic gastrointestinal disorders or surgery that results in chronic diarrhea are indications for additional vitamin and mineral supplementation.

3. T F Females require larger amounts of vitamins and minerals than males.

4. T F Vitamin A is processed from the carotene of plants and is a fat-soluble vitamin.

5. T F Vitamin K is synthesized in the body through the action of sunlight on the skin.

6. T F Fetal malformations have been reported following maternal ingestion of large doses of vitamin A, either before or during pregnancy.

7. T F Vitamin D is necessary for regulating the absorption and metabolism of calcium and phosphorus for healthy bones and teeth.

8. T F An overdose of vitamin D may antagonize with digoxin and thiazide diuretics.

9. T F Vitamin K is used for bleeding complications during the administration of heparin.

10. T F Vitamin B_6 (pyridoxine) is a coenzyme utilized in the metabolism of carbohydrates, fats, protein, and amino acids.

11. T F There is a significant increase in the foods high in vitamin B_6 after they have been frozen.

12. T F Vitamin B_{12} deficiency can be associated with patients on vegetarian diets or those who have a malabsorption syndrome.

13. T F The health care practitioner is aware that more than 50% of the supplemental dosage of vitamin C is excreted in the urine of normal subjects.

14. T F Patients should be encouraged to eat raw fresh fruits and vegetables for sources of vitamin C because heat and air destroy vitamin C.

15. T F Blood contains 90% sodium chloride, and the best source for oral intake of sodium chloride is table salt.

16. T F Hyperkalemia may cause a fall in the patient's blood pressure and/or cardiac arrhythmias.

17. T F The health care practitioner would instruct the patient in a calcium-rich diet to include vitamin D fortified whole milk, not low-fat milk.

18. T F When instructing the patient about taking oral iron preparations, the health care practitioner explains that nausea, vomiting, and other GI effects can be avoided by taking iron after or with meals but not with coffee, tea, or milk.

19. T F Iron should only be administered to patients with a confirmed diagnosis of deficiency through a blood test, and those with no peptic ulcer, regional enteritis, or ulcerative colitis.

20. T F Milk, cheese, and sardines are good sources of potassium.

Case Study

Georgia Reed, a 55-year-old woman, is diagnosed with pneumonia and dehydration. She has stated in her health history that she has had no intake for the last 2 days. Her physician has ordered an antibiotic for the pneumonia and 0.9% normal saline in 5% dextrose with 30 mEq KCL/liter @ 125 mL/h.

1. As the health care provider, which of the following data obtained from the patient would cause you concern related to the 30 mEq of KCL to be added to the IV fluids?

   A. Patient has not had any intake for 2 days.
   B. Patient states she has history of renal impairment.
   C. Patient's sister has diabetes.
   D. Patient complains of severe thirst.

2. The health care practitioner is aware that sodium and chloride are the principal minerals:

   A. Inside the body's cells.
   B. In 5% dextrose and water (D5W).
   C. In the extracellular body fluid.
   D. Rarely found in a normal adult diet.

3. The health care practitioner is attentive in that Georgia has not eaten in the last two days and that which of the following vitamins is likely depleted from her body because it is water soluble?

   A. Vitamin A
   B. Vitamin C
   C. Vitamin E
   D. Vitamin K

4. While Georgia is in the hospital, the pharmacist will prepare the IV fluids as follows:

   A. Add the 30 mEq KCL to the IV bag after it is started by the nurse.
   B. Administer 30 mEq KCL IV push first and then flush with the D5NS.
   C. Thoroughly mix the 30 mEq KCL in a liter bag of D5NS and run at 125 mL/h.
   D. Run at least 125 cc of D5NS, push the 30 mEq KCL, follow with D5NS at 125 mL/h.

5. The health care practitioner monitoring Georgia will be observing which of the following complications related to IV administration?

   A. Redness and heat around the infusion site.
   B. Leg pain.
   C. Increased urinary output.
   D. Heartburn.

CHAPTER 12

Skin Medications

Fill-in-the-Blank

Fill in the blank for each of the following statements.

1. The health care practitioner understands that a complete understanding of appropriate _____ for each topical medication is vital before administration.

2. Antipruritics are used short term to relieve discomfort from dermatitis related to allergic reactions, _____ _____ , hives, and insect bites.

3. Patients being treated with antipruritics should be instructed to first _____ the area thoroughly and then apply by gentle rubbing until the medication vanishes.

4. Corticosteroids are used both topically and _____ to treat dermatological disorders associated with allergic reactions.

5. For allergic reactions the antihistamine Benadryl is administered _____ for systemic effects.

6. Antihistamines applied topically in the form of lotion, cream, gel, or spray can cause _____ reactions and should only be used for a few days.

7. One of the side effects of long-term use of corticosteroid ointment or cream is increased fragility of cutaneous _____ _____ .

8. Use of corticosteroids is contraindicated in patients with bacterial or _____ skin infections and cutaneous or systemic viral infections.

9. Topical corticosteroids are also used to treat _____ and seborrheic dermatitis.

10. When a corticosteroid ointment or cream is used long term, a possible side effect is epidermal thinning, with frequent skin tears and increased risk of _____ and frequent _____ .

11. Demulcents and _____ are used topically to protect or soothe minor dermatological conditions, such as diaper rash, abrasions, and minor burns.

12. _____ agents are used to control conditions of abnormal scaling of the skin, such as dandruff, seborrhea, and psoriasis.

13. The topical enzyme collagenase (Santyl) should only be used on wounds associated with _____ tissue.

14. Lindane can be absorbed _____ following topical application and should be avoided during pregnancy and lactation, or with children and adults weighing less than 110 pounds.

15. Mycostatin oral suspension therapy for candidiasis should be administered to infants and adults following feedings and meals and after rinsing the _____ with water.

16. The health care practitioner should instruct the patient receiving treatment with an antifungal to follow application instructions carefully and use for the prescribed time, even if _____ subside.

17. For effective treatment of herpes zoster (shingles), Valtrex (a derivative of acyclovir) and Zovirax are oral _____ that need to be started within 72 hours of rash onset and are most effective if started within the first 48 hours of onset.

18. The two major antiseptics in use today are chlorhexidene and povidone-iodine, used for _____ scrubs and as _____ skin cleansers.

19. The health care practitioner is aware that chlorhexidene (Hibiclens) should not be used on wounds involving more than the _____ layers of skin and that it is important to rinse thoroughly after use.

20. If there is no improvement in a client's skin condition or the condition worsens or there are untoward reactions while using an antibacterial agent, the health care practitioner would advise the patient to _____ the medication and consult a _____ .

21. Accutane therapy is absolutely _____ in patients who are pregnant.

22. A patient taking Accutane for type 4 _____ may experience an altered lipid profile and a decrease in hemoglobin/hematocrit levels.

Multiple Choice

Circle the letter that best answers the question.

1. The health care practitioner is aware that the largest organ of the body is the:

   A. Skeletal.
   B. Lungs.
   C. Intestines.
   D. Skin.

2. The absorption of topical medications will be more rapid if the skin area is:

   A. Parched.
   B. Moist.
   C. Callused.
   D. Dehydrated.

3. Which of the following is a topical antipruritic medication?

   A. Coal tar
   B. Salicylic acid
   C. Sulfur
   D. Benzocaine

4. What is the generic name for Benadryl?

   A. Coal tar.
   B. Dibucaine.
   C. Diphenhydramine.
   D. Salicylic acid.

5. Which of the following is a topical keratolytic medication?

   A. Desitin
   B. Lindane
   C. Salicylic acid
   D. Mycostatin

6. Side effects of topical corticosteroids include

   A. Activation of latent infections and slow healing
   B. Photosensitivity and pruritus
   C. Temporary staining of the skin
   D. Arthralgia and myalgia

7. Which of these is the best description of scabies that a health care practitioner can give a patient?

   A. Another name for herpes zoster or shingles.
   B. Caused by an itch mite that burrows under the skin.
   C. A dermatitis associated with an allergic reaction such as poison ivy.
   D. Caused by an infestation of lice on the hairs of the scalp, pubic area, or trunk.

8. What should a health care practitioner teach a patient being treated with keratolytics about applying the prescribed medication?

   A. Only as long as the condition persists.
   B. Every other day for one week and every third day for the next week.
   C. Only as directed for the entire treatment period, even if the condition improves.
   D. For no more than one week, or if the condition improves do not restart.

9. In the treatment of pediculosis, which is a safer alternative to lindane?

   A. Pyrethrins
   B. Clortrimazole
   C. Acyclovir
   D. Chlorhexidene

10. Which of these provides the best explanation of pediculosis for a patient?

    A. Another name for herpes zoster or shingles.
    B. Caused by an itch mite that burrows under the skin.
    C. A dermatitis associated with an allergic reaction such as poison ivy.
    D. Caused by an infestation of lice on the hairs of the scalp, pubic area, or trunk.

11. When treating candidiasis of the oral cavity, how should Mycostatin oral suspension or oral lozenges be administered?

    A. Twice a day for 7 days.
    B. Three times a day for 10 days.
    C. Four times a day for 14 days.
    D. As needed and before meals.

12. Which of these statements about topical acyclovir therapy is correct?

    A. Decreases the duration of viral shedding, pain, and itching.
    B. Reduces the frequency and delays the appearance of new lesions.
    C. Keeps the lesions moist and prolongs crusting time.
    D. Is effective in preventing a secondary bacterial infection.

13. Substances that inhibit the growth of bacteria are called:

    A. Bactericidal.
    B. Disinfectant.
    C. Bacteriostatic.
    D. Antiviral.

14. Which of the following topical medications for burns would be ordered for a patient with an allergy to sulfa?

    A. Silvadene
    B. Hibiclens
    C. Lamisil
    D. Furacin

15. When applying topical medication to a burn, the health care practitioner should:

    A. Apply the medication with a sterile-gloved hand.
    B. Keep the burned area open after application.
    C. Apply the topical medication using a gauze pad and tongue blades.
    D. Spray the area, and leave it open.

16. Which of the following correctly describes pertinent education for the patient using an acne agent?

 A. Supplement retinoid agents with benzoyl peroxide application due to the possibility of scarring.
 B. Avoid multivitamins or nutritional supplements that contain vitamin A and the antacid aluminum hydroxide.
 C. Avoid use of sunscreen.
 D. Discontinue use if acne if not treated within a week of first application.

Matching A

Match the skin preparation in Column A with the action in Column B.

COLUMN A	COLUMN B
_____ 1. Antipruritic	A. Treat scabies
_____ 2. Emollients and demulcents	B. Prevent or treat infection of burned tissue
_____ 3. Keratolytic agents	C. Prevent and treat infection
_____ 4. Scabicides	D. Soothe irritation
_____ 5. Pediculicides	E. Control fungal conditions
_____ 6. Antifungals	F. Relieve itching
_____ 7. Local anti-infectives	G. Loosen epithelial scales
_____ 8. Antivirals	H. Treat herpes zoster
_____ 9. Silvadene	I. Treat lice

Matching B

Match the trade name of the topical medication in Column A with the generic name in Column B.

COLUMN A	COLUMN B
_____ 1. Clearasil	A. Acyclovir
_____ 2. Mycostatin	B. Zinc oxide
_____ 3. Neutrogena T/Gel	C. Salicylic acid
_____ 4. Desitin	D. Nystatin
_____ 5. Zovirax	E. Coal tar

True or False

Circle T for true or F for false after reading each of the following statements.

1. T   F   Keratolytic agents are used to promoted peeling of the skin in conditions such as acne, hard corns, calluses, and warts.

2. T   F   Emollients are contraindicated in immunosupressed patients and those who are presently receiving chemotherapy.

3. T   F   With prolonged use of high-potency corticosteroid products, patients may experience side effects such as hyperglycemia and Cushing's syndrome.

4. T   F   Lindane should be used only in patients who cannot tolerate or have failed first-line treatment with safer medications for the treatment of lice.

5. T   F   The oral dosage of Mycostatin for treatment of candidiasis should be used to coat the inside of the mouth and spit out as soon as possible.

6. T F The infant, child, or adult should be NPO for at least 1 hour after treatment with oral Mycostatin.

7. T F Patients being treated with antifungals should be instructed to expose the affected area to air whenever possible.

8. T F Topical therapy with the antiviral acyclovir is substantially more effective than systemic therapy (oral or parenteral).

9. T F There is an extremely high risk that birth defects can occur if pregnancy occurs while taking Accutane in any amount, even for a short period of time.

10. T F The absorption of topical medication is increased if the skin is thick and callused.

Case Study

A child in Mrs. White's kindergarten class was sent home with directions to see the family physician about the infestation of head lice. The physician has suggested that the child's hair be washed in RID and asked the health care practitioner in the office to instruct the parents in the treatment and care for the child with head lice.

1. As the health care provider, which of the following would you explain about the diagnosis of head lice?

   A. Head lice are similar to having athlete's feet except it is on the head.
   B. Head lice are caused by a virus and are transmitted through coughing.
   C. Head lice are easily transmitted from one person to the other by contact, either directly coming in contact with contaminated clothing or bed linens.
   D. When a rash develops due to itch mites burrowed under the skin, the medication must be started at that time.

2. The health care practitioner explains the use of RID as:

   A. A drug to take by mouth every 4 hours for 14 days.
   B. A body wash to clean the entire body with three times a day.
   C. A systemic treatment for the head lice to prevent spreading.
   D. A topical treatment in the form of a shampoo that will kill the lice.

3. In addition to the use of RID, for effective treatment of the head lice, which of the following instructions should be provided by the health care practitioner?

   A. Launder bedding in hot water or have it dry cleaned.
   B. Wash the child's clothing in cold water.
   C. Concurrent treatment for close contacts is usually not necessary.
   D. After beginning the treatment of RID, the child's head may be uncomfortable but the lice will be not easily transmitted.

4. The health care practitioner explains to the parents to stop using RID if which of the following occur?

   A. Any areas of the scalp become inflamed, raw, or begin to weep
   B. Sneezing several times after application
   C. The child complains of itching on the scalp
   D. The clothes the child was wearing that day are cleaned

Autonomic Nervous System Drugs

Fill-in-the-Blank

Fill in the blank for each of the following statements.

1. The autonomic nervous system is divided into the _sympathetic_ and the _parasympathetic_ divisions.

2. The autonomic nervous system is able to _____ respond to a person's needs.

3. The _sympathetic_ nervous system can be thought of as the emergency system used to rally the body for quick reaction and response.

4. Drugs that mimic the action of the sympathetic nervous system are called sympathomimetic or _____ .

5. Neurotransmitters released at the sympathetic nerve endings are called catecholamines and include _____, norepinephrine, and dopamine.

6. Because adrenergic drugs cause peripheral vasoconstriction and elevate the blood pressure, they are used in all types of _____.

7. Adrenergic drugs are sometimes applied topically to relieve nosebleed due to their action of capillary _____ .

8. Health care practitioners should caution patients beginning on a beta-adrenergic blocking agent to rise slowly from a reclining position to avoid postural _____ .

9. Patients taking beta-adrenergic blocking agents should be taught that sexual dysfunction or depression should be reported to the physician for possible dosage _____ or change to a different medication.

10. Parasympathomimetic or _____ drugs mimic the action of the parasympathetic nervous system.

11. Drugs that block the action of the parasympathetic nervous system are called cholinergic blockers or _____ .

12. Parasympatholytics most commonly used as preoperative medications include _____ and glycopyrrolate (Robinul).

13. For patients who have chronic obstructive pulmonary disease (COPD), _____ type inhalations of aerosols are recommended.

14. When administering cholinergic blocking agents with an antihistamine such as diphenhydramine, _____ of sedation and drying effects can occur.

15. Anticholinergics are sometimes used as antidotes for insecticide or _____ poisoning, or cholinergic crisis.

16. Confusion and/or excitement are possible side effects of cholinergic blocking agents, particularly when administered to _____ _____ .

17. Anticholinergics are often ordered for patients with abdominal pain due to their potential for decreasing gastrointestinal _____ and gastric secretions.

18. Health care practitioners should instruct patients with chronic obstructive lung disease and asthma to _____ use of oral or over-the-counter anticholinergics, and only use anticholinergics ordered by their physician.

Multiple Choice

Circle the letter that best answers the question.

1. Chemical substances released at the sympathetic and parasympathetic nerve endings that modify or result in the spread of nerve impulses are called:

   A. Analgesics.
   B. Neurotransmitters.
   C. Anticholinergics.
   D. Adrenergics.

2. The sympathomimetic drugs mimic the action of the sympathetic nervous system which causes an increase in:

   A. Contraction of the urinary bladder.
   B. Peristalsis.
   C. Saliva production.
   D. Blood pressure.

3. Drugs that mimic the action of the parasympathetic nervous system, are called parasympathomimetics or:

   A. Cholinergics.
   B. Adrenergics.
   C. Cholinergic blockers.
   D. Adrenergic blockers.

4. What is the primary outcome of the adrenergic drug administered to patients experiencing an acute asthma attack or an anaphylactic reaction?

   A. Slowing peristalsis.
   B. Peripheral vasodilatation.
   C. Dilating bronchioles.
   D. Dilation of the pupils.

5. Adrenergic medications should be administered with extreme caution and are sometimes contraindicated in patients with:

   A. Hypotension.
   B. Normal kidney function.
   C. Coronary insufficiency.
   D. Bradycardia.

6. The health care practitioner should observe a patient receiving an adrenergic medication for which of these side effects?

   A. Hyperglycemia, tachycardia, nervousness, and anginal pain.
   B. Hypotension, bradycardia, hypoglycemia, and confusion.
   C. Muscle cramps, weakness, and constriction of the pupils.
   D. Jaundice, hypotension, and sweating.

7. Adrenergic blockers are those medications that block the action of the sympathetic nervous system and are commonly called:

   A. Monoamine oxidase inhibitors.
   B. Tricyclic antidepressants.
   C. Cardiac glycosides.
   D. Beta blockers.

8. Which of these drugs is considered to be the prototype of beta-adrenergic blockers?

    A. Inderal.
    B. Levophed.
    C. Isuprel.
    D. Atropine.

9. A health care practitioner should observe a patient receiving an adrenergic blocking agent for which of these side effects?

    A. Hyperglycemia, tachycardia, nervousness, and anginal pain.
    B. Hypotension, bradycardia, hypoglycemia, and fatigue.
    C. Muscle cramps, weakness, and euphoria.
    D. Jaundice, hypertension, and sweating.

10. Adrenergic blockers should be administered with extreme caution and are sometimes contraindicated in patients with:

    A. Migraine headache.
    B. Hypertension.
    C. Congestive heart failure.
    D. Angina pectoris.

11. Which of these actions should be taught to patients taking adrenergic blocking agents?

    A. Take medication at least once to twice a week as needed.
    B. Keep medication on hand in case their blood pressure goes up.
    C. Not to discontinue the medication abruptly, except on the advice of their physician.
    D. Take medication for 2 weeks and stop for 2 weeks.

12. Parasympathetic nerve fibers produce and release which neurotransmitter at their postganglionic nerve endings as the mediator?

    A. Norephinephrine
    B. Acetylcholine
    C. Epinephrine
    D. Dopamine

13. Actions of cholinergic drugs include which of the following?

    A. Tachycardia, pupil dilation, and dry mouth
    B. Decreased contraction of the urinary bladder
    C. Lowered intraocular pressure and increased gastrointestinal motility
    D. Cardiac stimulation, bronchodilation, and increased blood to skeletal muscles

14. Pilocarpine ophthalmic drops are cholinergic drugs which are prescribed to

    A. Lower intraocular pressure with glaucoma.
    B. Increase contraction of the bladder with benign prostatic hypertrophy.
    C. Improve the symptoms of hyperthyroidism.
    D. Improve vision in patients with cataracts.

15. Which anticholinergic medication reduces the incidence of laryngospasm and acts as a bronchodilator during general anesthesia?

    A. Scopolamine
    B. Homatropine
    C. Robinul
    D. Atropine

16. Anticholinergic medication such as the Atrovent inhaler is used in the prevention and treatment of:

    A. Bronchospasm.
    B. Spastic gastrointestinal disorders.
    C. Dilation of pupils.
    D. Emergency treatment of bradycardia.

17. Pro-Banthine, a parasympatholytic drug, is used in the treatment of:

    A. Bronchospasm.
    B. Bladder spasm.
    C. Dilation of pupils.
    D. Bradycardia.

18. What common medication ordered for motion sickness is a cholinergic blocker?

    A. Urecholine.
    B. Inderal.
    C. Scopolamine.
    D. Aramine.

19. Anticholinergics are ordered as preoperative medications because they

    A. Increase gastrointestinal peristalsis
    B. Lower intraocular pressure
    C. Dry secretions and prevent hypotension and bradycardia
    D. Increase gastric secretions and prevent muscle cramps and constipation

20. Which of the following side effects would the health care practitioner observe for in a patient receiving an anticholinergic agent?

    A. Blurred vision, headache, dry mouth, palpitations, and tachycardia
    B. Hypotension, bradycardia, cholinergic crisis, and fatigue
    C. Muscle cramps, weakness, and euphoria
    D. Jaundice, excessive salivation, and sweating

Matching

Match the category of autonomic nervous system drugs listed in Column A with the action or use of the drugs in the specific category in Column B. Note that the choices in Column B can be used more than once.

COLUMN A	COLUMN B
_____ 1. Lower blood pressure	A. Adrenergics
_____ 2. Bronchodilation	B. Cholinergics
___ 3. Angina pectoris	C. Beta-adrenergic blockers
_____ 4. Cardiac stimulation	D. Cholinergic blockers
_____ 5. Increased peristalsis	
_____ 6. Increased secretions	
_____ 7. Drying (all secretions decreased)	
_____ 8. Dilation of pupils	
_____ 9. Migraine headaches	
_____ 10. Peripheral vasoconstriction	
_____ 11. Increased contraction of the urinary bladder	
_____ 12. Increased flow to skeletal muscles	
_____ 13. Cardiac arrhythmias	
_____ 14. Constriction of pupils	
_____ 15. Slowing of the heart	
_____ 16. Decreased GI and GU motility	
_____ 17. Constriction of pupils	
_____ 18. Decrease in intraocular pressure	

True or False

Circle T for true or F for false after reading each of the following statements.

1. T F Key words used to describe the parasympathetic nervous system are fright, fight, and flight.

2. T F Adrenergics are sometimes combined with local anesthetics to constrict capillaries and decrease bleeding during minor surgery.

3. T F Epinephrine is an adrenergic blocking agent that lowers the blood pressure when taken consistently.

4. T F Adrenergic agents are often administered to patients for ophthalmic procedures because of their mydriatic action.

5. T F The adrenergic blocker propranolol is used for patients with angina, arrhythmias, and for migraine headaches.

6. T F Health care practitioners must teach patients taking a beta-adrenergic blocking agent that interactions could occur if they are also taking theophylline, digoxin, insulin, or oral antidiabetic agents.

7. T F Respiratory depression is a side effect of cholinergic drugs and may result in a cholinergic crisis.

8. T F Patients with gastric ulcers are appropriate candidates to receive cholinergic drugs such as neostigmine.

9. T F Anticholinergics increase the motility of the gastrointestinal tract and the genitourinary system.

10. T F Homatropine ophthalmic drops are classified as an anticholinergic medication used to dilate the pupils.

Case Study

Sally Reed, 45 years old, attends the medical clinic once every month. She always brings her medications with her for review. Sally was diagnosed with myasthenia gravis last year and the clinic doctors are still trying to get her medications regulated. This is the first time this health care practitioner has assessed Sally prior to her visit with the physician. While Sally is waiting for the physician, she asks the health care practitioner about the side effects of her medications.

1. When caring for Sally for the first time, the health care practitioner should question which of the following combinations of drugs due to possible interaction?

    A. Prostigmin and quinidine
    B. Urecholine and Tylenol
    C. Tensilon and Colace
    D. Pilocarpine and Zantac

2. The health care practitioner is aware that the type of medications that mimic the neurotransmitter acetylcholine is parasympathomimetics or:

    A. Adrenergics.
    B. Cholinergics.
    C. Beta-adrenergic blockers.
    D. Cholinergic blockers.

3. The health care practitioner explains the following side effects of her medication for myasthenia gravis (parasympathomimetics) as:

    A. Tachycardia, nervousness, and anginal pain.
    B. Constipation and pale skin color.
    C. Nausea, vomiting, muscle cramps, weakness, and low blood pressure.
    D. Jaundice, hypertension, euphoria, decreased sweating.

4. The health care practitioner recalls the diagnoses for which parasympathomimetics are contraindicated such as:

   A. Intestinal obstruction.
   B. Hyperthyroidism.
   C. Glaucoma.
   D. Bronchitis.

5. The health care practitioner knows that the treatment for acute toxicity or cholinergic crisis is:

   A. IV atropine sulfate.
   B. PO urecholine.
   C. Pilocarpine eyedrops.
   D. IV tensilon.

CHAPTER 14

Antineoplastic Drugs

Fill-in-the-Blank

Fill in the blank for each of the following statements.

1. Antineoplastic agents counteract the development, growth, or spread of _____ _____ .

2. Cytotoxic drugs administered for cancer chemotherapy typically cause the death of proliferating cells or those that reproduce _____ .

3. The proliferating cells destroyed by cytotoxic drugs consist of not only cancerous cells but also many normal proliferating tissues such as _____ _____ , gastrointestinal epithelium, skin, hair follicles, and epithelium of the gonads.

4. Numerous _____ side effects occur with the use of antineoplastic drugs.

5. A common toxic effect of antineoplastic agents is to decrease the production of antibodies and phagocytes and _____ the patient's inflammatory reaction.

6. Targeted therapies are a significant development in antineoplastic drugs such as monoclonal _____ , which are designed to target only cancer cells and spare normal tissues.

7. Suppression of the immune response results in increased _____ of the patient to infection.

8. Cytotoxic drugs are administered in very high doses but usually on an _____ schedule, allowing normal cells to repair during the drug-free time.

9. Careful planning is necessary to maximize the _____ of chemotherapy and minimize the adverse effects and discomfort for the patient.

10. Patients taking antimetabolites should be aware that this treatment may result in alopecia and that regrowth of hair may take several _____ after concluding treatment.

11. As with many antineoplastics, patients receiving antimetabolites will likely experience bone marrow suppression, including leucopenia, _____ , and thrombocytopenia.

12. Patients receiving _____ agents need to be aware that this treatment may cause the loss of reproductive capacity.

13. The patient receiving intravenous vinblastine, a mitotic inhibitor, will likely experience tissue _____ if the IV solution infiltrates into the tissue.

14. Miotic inhibitors must never be administered to patients via the intrathecal route because they are _____ when given intrathecally.

15. With the administration of paclitaxel (Taxol), hypersensitivity reactions can be severe, including flushing, rash, _____ , chest pain, hypotension, and bradycardia.

16. Because paclitaxel (Taxol) is so toxic, it is only administered IV under continuous supervision of an _____ , with frequent monitoring of vital signs and facilities on hand for emergency interventions if necessary.

17. Anti-tumor antineoplastic agents are frequently used in _____ with other drugs and ordered to treat a wide variety of malignancies.

18. The antitumor antibiotics often have the side effect of _____ _____ suppression.

19. Side effects such as fluid retention, cushingoid features, fatigue and weakness, and osteoporosis are common with prolonged use of _____ such as Prednisone.

20. An oral antiandrogen, _____ , is used simultaneously with leuprolide in the treatment of metastatic prostate cancer.

21. A class of monoclonal antibodies are _____ , genetically engineered in the laboratory.

22. Monoclonal antibodies are designed to target only _____ cells.

23. Monoclonal antibodies reduce _____ toxicity while increasing toxicity to cancer cells.

24. The monoclonal antibody Avastin, used in combination with fluorouracil, is indicated for first-line treatment of patients with _____ carcinoma of the colon or rectum.

25. Severe reactions to monoclonal antibodies can be decreased by _____ with acetaminophen, diphenhydramine, and/or meperidine.

26. Radioactive material is sometimes implanted in the patient's body in the form of capsules, needles, or _____ .

27. Health care practitioners must observe special precautions when caring for patients receiving _____ _____ to prevent unnecessary radiation exposure.

28. Intravenous sites must be checked with great care because antineoplastic agents can cause extreme tissue damage and necrosis if _____ occurs.

29. Intravenous fluids containing antineoplastic agents must not get on skin or into the _____ of the patient or health care provider administering the fluids.

30. It is most important for health care practitioners to be knowledgeable about the common side effects of antineoplastic drugs interventions, _____ , and appropriate patient education.

Multiple Choice

Circle the letter that best answers the question.

1. Antineoplastic drugs are cytotoxic or destructive to cells, especially those cells that are:

   A. Rapidly dividing.
   B. In the resting stage.
   C. Dormant.
   D. Inactive.

2. Newer antineoplastic treatments that specifically target cancer cells and avoid severe toxicity to normal cells are called:

   A. Radioactive isotopes.
   B. Hormones.
   C. Monoclonal antibodies.
   D. Antimetabolites.

3. The choice of chemotherapeutic agents in combination drug therapy is based upon which of these factors?

   A. age of patient
   B. source of the cancer
   C. cost of drugs to be used
   D. type of malignancy

4. Antimetabolites should be administered with extreme caution and/or are sometimes contraindicated in patients with:

   A. Leukemia.
   B. Breast cancer.
   C. Renal and hepatic disorders.
   D. Lupus and rheumatoid arthritis.

5. What drug, a reduced form of folic acid, is sometimes used as a rescue agent following methotrexate administration to reduce side effects of methotrexate?

   A. Prednisone
   B. Leucovorin
   C. Mesna
   D. Taxol

6. Patients with bone marrow suppression experiencing thrombocytopenia will have the risk of:

   A. Hemorrhage.
   B. Infection.
   C. Coronary insufficiency.
   D. Bradycardia.

7. Patients with bone marrow suppression experiencing leukopenia will be at risk for:

   A. Hyperglycemia.
   B. Hypotension.
   C. Infection.
   D. Hemorrhage.

8. A patient experiencing neurotoxicity as a side effect of receiving alkylating agents would have which of these symptoms?

   A. Sore throat, dry mouth, and cough
   B. Nausea, vomiting, and diarrhea
   C. Headache, vertigo, and seizures
   D. Chest pain, vomiting, and dry mouth

9. What is the chemoprotectant given prior to the alkylating agent ifosfamide to prevent hemorrhagic cystitis?

   A. Leucovorin
   B. Mesna
   C. Cisplatin
   D. Atropine

10. Which of these antineoplastic agents is contraindicated in patients with renal disease?

    A. Taxol
    B. Tamoxifen
    C. Cisplatin
    D. Cobalt

11. What symptoms of neurotoxicity would the patient experience as a side effect of receiving the plant alkaloid vincristine?

    A. Numbness, tingling, ataxia
    B. Tachycardia, pupil dilation, and dry mouth
    C. Bronchospasm and urinary frequency
    D. Infection of the IV site and necrosis of the tissue

12. Which corticosteroid administered in large doses prior to or along with chemotherapy has been found effective in the prevention and management of nausea and vomiting associated with neoplastic agents?

    A. Prednisone
    B. Dexamethasone
    C. Leucovorin
    D. Tamoxifen

13. Which corticosteroid is used in combination with other chemotherapeutic agents to help prevent severe allergic reactions?

    A. Prednisone
    B. Arimidex
    C. Leucovorin
    D. Tamoxifen

14. What nonsteroidal antiestrogen is used as primary hormonal therapy for metastatic estrogen receptor-positive breast cancer in both men and postmenopausal women?

    A. Decadron.
    B. Daunorubicin.
    C. Tamoxifen.
    D. Prednisone.

15. Which antiandrogen drug is administered once monthly IM for prostate cancer?

    A. Tamoxifen
    B. Casodex
    C. Leuprolide acetate
    D. Prednisone

16. Which of these agents is a complex combination of many proteins that boost immune system response?

    A. Interferon alfa.
    B. Dexamethasone.
    C. Radioactive isotopes.
    D. Antibiotics.

17. Which monoclonal antibodies are used in combination with fluorouracil as a first-line treatment of patients with metastatic carcinoma of the colon or rectum?

    A. Rituxin
    B. Avastin
    C. Herceptin
    D. Arimidex

18. Which monoclonal antibodies are used in combination with paclitaxel as a first-line treatment of patients with metastatic breast cancer?

    A. Rituxin
    B. Avastin
    C. Herceptin
    D. Arimidex

19. All monoclonal antibodies are administered by which route?

    A. Oral
    B. Intramuscular
    C. Intravenous
    D. Intrathecal

20. Zofran, Anzemet, and Kytril are all examples of medications used in conjunction with antineoplastic drugs in order to treat, minimize, or prevent:

    A. Ulcers in the mouth.
    B. Infections.
    C. Numbness and tingling of the extremities.
    D. Nausea and vomiting.

Matching A

Match the key term in Column A with its definition in Column B.

COLUMN A	COLUMN B
_____ 1. Antineoplastic	A. Substance or procedure that reduces or prevents an immune response
_____ 2. Chemotherapy	B. Increase or multiplication of cells rapidly
_____ 3. Cytotoxic	C. Alleviation of symptoms
_____ 4. Immunosuppressive	D. Cytotoxic drugs and drug combinations used to destroy cancer cells
_____ 5. Palliative	E. Destructive to cells
_____ 6. Proliferate	F. Agent that counteracts the development, growth, and spread of malignant cells

Matching B

Match the neoplastic agent in Column A with the classification in Column B.

COLUMN A	COLUMN B
_____ 1. Vincristine	A. Antimetabolites
_____ 2. Paclitaxel	B. Alkylating agents
_____ 3. Cisplatin	C. Mitotic inhibitors
_____ 4. Prednisone	D. Antitumor antibiotics
_____ 5. Bleomycin	E. Corticosteroid
_____ 6. Leucovorin	F. Antiestrogen
_____ 7. Interferon alfa	G. Oral antiandrogen
_____ 8. Radiogold	H. IM antiandrogen
_____ 9. Tamoxifen	I. Immununotherapies
_____ 10. Leuprolide acetate	J. Rescue agent
_____ 11. Fluorouracil	K. Radioactive isotopes
_____ 12. Bicalutamide	
_____ 13. Methotrexate	

True or False

Circle T for true or F for false after reading each of the following statements.

1. T F Cancer therapy frequently includes a combination of surgery, radiation, and/or chemotherapy.

2. T F The new treatment for cancer using monoclonal antibodies is designed to spare normal tissues and only target cancer cells.

3. T F Chemotherapy is given exactly on the same schedule with each patient in order to get the best result from the antineoplastic agents.

4. T F Carmustine is an antimetabolite often administered to patients for resistant cases of rheumatoid arthritis.

5. T F Alkylating agents are used in the treatment of patients with brain tumors, sarcomas, lymphomas, and leukemias.

6. T F Patients with leukemia, Hodgkin's disease, lymphomas, and sarcomas may receive mitotic inhibitors like vincristine and vinblastine.

7. T F Cardiotoxicity, including arrhythmias and congestive heart failure, are side effects of the antineoplastic antibiotics bleomycin and mitomycin.

8. T F Patients receiving prednisone over a prolonged period of time have been found to have no major side effects.

9. T F Side effects of the antiestrogen tamoxifen resemble menopausal symptoms such as nausea, vomiting, hot flashes, and night sweats.

10. T F Side effects of antiandrogens include impotence, generalized pain, infection, constipation, and nausea.

11. T F Adverse side effects of interferons include flulike symptoms, anorexia, dry mouth, transient alopecia, leukopenia, and sleep or mental disturbances.

12. T F Monoclonal antibodies are designed to target only cancer cells.

13. T F Side effects of monoclonal antibodies are common and get progressively worse with each treatment.

14. T F Severe reactions occurring with the administration of monoclonal antibodies include angioedema, hypotension, dyspnea, bronchospasm, and anaphylaxis.

15. T F Radioactive sodium iodine is administered PO or IV to treat thyroid cancer.

16. T F The primary side effect of radioimmunotherapy is a decreased blood count occurring 4–6 weeks after treatment, with a duration of 2–3 weeks.

17. T F The distinct advantage of radioimmunotherapy is that it is typically given one time.

18. T F Aseptic technique is necessary to minimize the chance of infection in patients receiving antineoplastics drugs due to their reduced resistance to infection.

Case Study

Ed Rome, a 67-year-old patient, just arrived at the oncology outpatient clinic to receive a dose of chemotherapy for bladder cancer. This is the second time he has received the antineoplastic agent, 5-fluorouracil. Mr. Rome complained of "ulcers in his mouth." The health care provider checks the patient's blood work completed the previous day. She then prepares to administer his chemotherapy.

1. In which classification of antineoplastics is 5-fluorouracil included?

  A. Antimetabolite.
  B. Alkylating agent.
  C. Mitotic inhibitor.
  D. Anti-tumor antibiotic.

2. The health care provider should assess the patient's blood work for which of these?

   A. Photosensitivity
   B. Bone marrow suppression
   C. Pulmonary fibrosis
   D. Impotence

3. In order to decrease the amount of nausea and vomiting associated with 5-fluorouracil, the physician will likely order an antiemetic such as:

   A. Bleomycin.
   B. Daunorubicin.
   C. Zofran.
   D. Tensilon.

4. What information should the health care provider include when teaching the patient and family?

   A. Side effects are probably minimal with this antineoplastic.
   B. Careful oral hygiene with a soft toothbrush to prevent further trauma to ulcerated mucosa.
   C. No dietary restrictions are necessary.
   D. Making arrangements with hospice services as soon as possible.

Urinary System Drugs

Fill-in-the-Blank

Fill in the blank for each of the following statements.

1. The type of diuretic ordered by the physician is determined by the _condition_ being treated.

2. Thiazide diuretics are ordered for _sever_ hypertension to reduce peripheral resistance and decrease fluid retention.

3. Because thiazide diuretics increase the excretion of water, sodium, chloride and _potassium_, they are used to decrease edema from many causes such as heart failure.

4. Common side effects of the thiazide diuretics include _hypokalemia_ (potassium deficiency) and _hyponatremia_ (low serum sodium.)

5. Patients taking thiazide diuretics on a regular basis should be taught to include potassium-rich foods such as _bananas_ and citrus fruits in their diet due to the potential of potassium deficiency.

6. Thiazide diuretics must be used with great caution in patients with a history of gout, impaired liver disease, and severe _renal_ disease.

7. The health care practitioner should teach the patient taking a thiazide diuretic to rise slowly to prevent severe episodes of _postural hypotension_

8. Reabsorption of sodium and chloride on the loop of Henle in the kidney is inhibited by _loop_ diuretics.

9. Side effects of loop diuretics include _headace_, muscle cramps, dizziness, and mental confusion.

10. The potential for digoxin _____ and arrhythmias is increased when digoxin is and loop diuretics are taken simultaneously.

11. When furosemide is taken concurrently with an anticonvulsant, the diuretic effect of the furosemide is _reduce_ .

12. Mannitol is used to promote _excresion_ of toxins.

13. Kidney and _heart_ function should be evaluated before administration of osmotic agents to anyone with kidney failure, heart failure, or severe pulmonary edema.

14. The patient receiving mannitol should be reassured that osmotic agents are always given under close medical supervision, and serum _electrolytes_ will be monitored frequently by blood tests to detect adverse reactions.

15. Medications used to treat chronic gout include uricosuric agents and allopurinol, which lower _uric acid_ levels.

16. During acute attacks of gout, patients are treated with colchicine for its anti-inflammatory actions to supplement the uricosuric agent such as probenecid, which blocks _reabsorption_ and promotes urinary excretion of uric acid.

76

17. The uricosuric agent ___probencid___ is sometimes used with antibiotics to potentiate the blood level of the antibiotic.

18. For patients who have chronic gout, _____ is ordered because it decreases urine levels of uric acid by inhibiting an enzyme responsible for the production of uric acid, resulting in decreased serum uric acid levels.

19. The antispasmodics Ditropan and Detrol are used for relief of symptoms of urgency, frequency, ___nocturia___, and incontinence.

20. All antispasmodics that are anticholingeric in action should be used cautiously in ___older adults___ because adverse side effects are common in this patient population.

21. Patients taking anticholinergic antispasmodics commonly complain of dryness of secretions, particularly in the mouth and ___eyes___ .

22. Anticholinergic antispasmodics are ___contraindicated___ in children under 5 years of age.

23. The cholinogeric drug ___Bethanechol___ (Urecholine) has been called the "pharmacological catheterization."

24. The oral urinary analgesic phenazopyridine (Pyridium) is used only for ___symptomatic___ relief of burning, pain, and urgency associated with cystitis.

25. Benign prostatic hypertrophy (BPH) can be treated with medications such as antiandrogens or ___alpha___ blockers.

Multiple Choice

Circle the letter that best answers the question.

1. Which classification of diuretics are most frequently ordered by physicians?

   A. Loop
   B. Osmotic
   C. Potassium-sparing
   D. Thiazide

2. Furosemide and bumetanide are examples of which type of diuretics?

   A. Thiazide
   B. Potassium-sparing
   C. Loop
   D. Osmotic

3. Which type of diuretic will usually used to treat a patient suffering from pulmonary edema or edema associated with impaired renal function or hepatic function?

   A. Loop, e.g., Lasix
   B. Osmotic, e.g., mannitol
   C. Potassium-sparing, e.g., Aldactone
   D. Thiazide, e.g., hydrochlorothiazide

4. Side effects of bumetanide and furosemide include:

   A. Hypokalemia with weakness and vertigo.
   B. Hypertension and GI effects.
   C. Hypoglycemia and decreased uric acid levels.
   D. Fluid and electrolyte imbalance such as overhydration.

5. Loop diuretics are contraindicated or used with caution in patients who have:

   A. Hypertension.
   B. Allergy to penicillin.
   C. A history of cirrhosis of the liver.
   D. Kidney impairment.

6. Aldactazide and Dyazide are classified as which category of diuretics?

   A. Thiazide
   B. Loop
   C. Potassium-sparing
   D. Combination potassium-sparing and thiazide

7. When administering the cardiac drug digoxin along with loop diuretics, the health care practitioner is aware that there is a potential for:

   A. The heart rate to speed up to a dangerous level.
   B. Digitalis toxicity and arrhythmias to occur.
   C. The pupils to dilate.
   D. Skin to appear jaundiced.

8. The health care practitioner is aware that gynecomastia is a side effect of which of the following diuretics?

   A. Lasix
   B. Allopurinol
   C. Probenecid
   D. Spironolactone

9. When administering potassium-sparing diuretics to patients who also take medications such as ACE inhibitors, NSAIDs, angiotensin receptor blockers, and salicylates, the health care practitioner should be aware that which of these interactions may occur?

   A. Hypokalemia.
   B. Hyperkalemia.
   C. Pulmonary edema.
   D. Hyperglycemia.

10. The osmotic agent mannitol is most frequently used to:

    A. Treat pulmonary edema.
    B. Lower blood pressure.
    C. Reduce intracranial or intraocular pressure.
    D. Promote diuresis in patients with cirrhosis.

11. Which diuretic interacts to increase urinary excretion of other medications, lowering blood levels of lithium, salicylates, and barbiturates?

    A. Aldactone
    B. Aldactazide
    C. Lasix
    D. Mannitol

12. Which of these diuretics is administered only via the parenteral route?

    A. Aldactone
    B. Furosemide
    C. Mannitol
    D. Spironolactone

13. When a patient is taking a combination potassium-sparing and thiazide diuretic, the health care practitioner should emphasize the need for

    A. consuming the medication with meals
    B. consuming the medication at bedtime
    C. periodic serum electrolyte checks
    D. weighing self several times a day

14. Which of these diuretics can be administered via the PO, IM, or IV routes?

    A. Thiazide diuretics
    B. Loop diuretics
    C. Potassium-sparing diuretics
    D. Osmotic agents

15. Uricosuric agents and allopurinol are used only to treat chronic gout because they

    A. have no analgesic or anti-inflammatory effects in acute gout.
    B. are poorly absorbed and do not relieve the symptoms of acute gout.
    C. are not effective in producing diuresis.
    D. have no effect in reducing the uric acid levels.

16. Which of these actions should the health care practitioner include when teaching patients who are receiving uricosuric agents?

    A. Take aspirin as needed to control pain.
    B. Take the uricosuric agent 2 to 3 hours after meals to avoid nausea and vomiting.
    C. Drink large amounts of fluid, preferably water, to avoid kidney stones and renal colic.
    D. Carefully observe for any signs of hyperglycemia.

17. Which medications used for chronic gout is also used to prevent renal calculi in patients with history of frequent stone formation, and prevent acute hyperuricemia during radiation of certain tumors or antineoplastic therapy?

    A. Allopurinol
    B. Bethanechol
    C. Oxbutynin
    D. Propantheline

18. Antispasmodics such as propantheline are used to reduce the strength and frequency of contractions of the urinary bladder by:

    A. Stimulating parasympathetic nerve impulses.
    B. Blocking parasympathetic nerve impulses.
    C. Stimulating sympathetic nerve impulses.
    D. Blocking alpha-1 receptors in smooth muscles.

19. The side effects of antispasmodics are anticholinergic in action and can include which of the following?

    A. Hypotension, bradycardia, and bladder contraction
    B. Sweating, salivation, and GI cramping
    C. Excessive secretions from mucous membranes
    D. Urinary retention and mental confusion, especially in older adults

Matching A

Match the drug in Column A with the category in Column B. Note that the choices in Column B can be used more than once.

COLUMN A	COLUMN B
_____ 1. Bumetanide	A. Thiazide diuretics
_____ 2. Maxzide	B. Loop diuretics
_____ 3. Aldactazide	C. Potassium-sparing diuretics
_____ 4. Mannitol	D. Combination potassium-sparing and thiazide diuretics
_____ 5. Demadex	E. Osmotic agents

(*Matching continued on next page*)

COLUMN A
(continued)

_____ 6. Aldactone

_____ 7. Hydrochlorothiazide

_____ 8. Zaroxolyn

_____ 9. Lasix

Matching B

Match the terms describing unexpected responses to drugs in Column A with the description of the term in Column B.

COLUMN A	COLUMN B
_____ 1. Teratogenic	A. Severe hypersensitivity response, possibly requiring CPR; may be fatal allergic reaction
_____ 2. Idiosyncrasy	B. Immune response to a drug may be of varying degrees
_____ 3. Paradoxical	C. Effect from maternal drug administration that causes the development of physical defects in a fetus
_____ 4. Tolerance	D. Acquired need for a drug that may produce psychological and/ or physical symptoms of withdrawal when the drug is discontinued
_____ 5. Dependence	E. Unique, unusual response to a drug
_____ 6. Hypersensitivity	F. Decreased response to a drug that develops after repeated doses are given
_____ 7. Anaphylactic reaction	G. Opposite effect from the drug that was expected

True or False

Circle T for true or F for false after reading each of the following statements.

1. T F Administering thiazide and loop diuretics along with corticosteroids may lead to an increased potassium loss.

2. T F The action of loop diuretics is more rapid and effective than thiazide diuretics with greater diuresis.

3. T F Potassium-sparing diuretics counteract the increased glucose and uric acid levels associated with thiazide diuretic therapy.

4. T F Patients being treated with furosemide should be taught to spend time in the sun to improve the therapeutic effect.

5. T F The diuretic of choice for patients with cirrhosis of the liver is spironolactone; however, it should still be used with caution.

6. T F Hyperkalemia may be a side effect of potassium-sparing diuretics such as dyrenium.

7. T F Patients receiving potassium-sparing diuretics should be instructed to avoid potassium-rich foods and salt substitutes.

8. T F Osmotic agents such as mannitol are administered by mouth or intravenously.

9. T F Probenecid, a uricosuric agent used for chronic gout, is also given with cefoxitin to treat acute pelvic inflammatory disease because it potentiates the therapeutic effect of antibiotics.

10. T F Severe hypersensitivity reactions with the medication allopurinol are rare but increase in patients with renal impairment who receive a combination of allopurinol and thiazide diuretics.

11. T F   A patient taking allopurinol should be encouraged to drink alcohol daily in order to potentiate the decrease in the amount of uric acid produced.

12. T F   Extended release formulations such as ditropan XL may cause fewer anticholinergic adverse effects than other antispasmodics.

Case Study

Peg Whitaker, a 62-year-old woman, is diagnosed with hypertension and has a history of congestive heart failure. Her physician has ordered a diuretic and 0.125 mg of digoxin every day.

1. The health care practitioner is aware that which one of the following diuretics is the first line for uncomplicated hypertension?

   A. Mannitol
   B. Furosemide
   C. Hydrochlorothiazide
   D. Dyazide

2. When should the health care practitioner instruct Peg to take her diuretic?

   A. Just before bedtime.
   B. With food in the morning.
   C. 2 hours after lunch.
   D. 1 hour before the evening meal.

3. The health care practitioner will also encourage Peg to include foods in her diet that are rich in:

   A. Sodium.
   B. Magnesium.
   C. Phosphorus.
   D. Potassium.

4. If Peg should have an acute episode of congestive heart failure in the future, which diuretic will the physician most likely order?

   A. Mannitol
   B. Furosemide
   C. Hydrochlorothiazide
   D. Aldactazide

Gastrointestinal Drugs

Fill-in-the-Blank

Fill in the blank for each of the following statements.

1. Antacids partially neutralize gastric _hydrochloric acid_ for relief of indigestion, heartburn, and sour stomach.

2. Antacids should not be taken within _two_ _hours_ of most other drugs because they can either increase or decrease absorption of other medications.

3. When diazepam is administered with antacids, the _sedative_ effect of diazepam is _increase_.

4. When amphetamines and quinidine are administered with antacids, cardiac irregularities are _uncreased_.

5. The effectiveness of digoxin, indomethacin, and iron is _decreased_ when administered with antacids.

6. The antiulcer drugs _Tagemet_ and _zantac_ are most likely to have interactions with other medications such as phenytoin, diazepam, theophylline, and tricyclic antidepressants.

7. A synthetic form of prostaglandin E_1, called _Misoprostol_, inhibits gastric acid secretion and protects the mucosa from the irritant effect of drugs such as NSAIDs.

8. Older adult patients who use drugs that reduce gastric acid on a long-term basis by are at risk of depleting the _____ _____ necessary for absorption of vitamin B_{12}.

9. Dicyclomine should be _____ in patients taking phenothiazines and tricyclic antidepressants because it alters the effects of these medications.

10. The health care practitioner should instruct patients undergoing therapy for ulcers that cigarette smoking _decrease_ the effectiveness of medicines in the healing of duodenal ulcers.

11. The health care practitioner should instruct patients to restructure their environment to reduce stress factors and _decrease_ tension to facilitate the healing of ulcers and reduce gastric motility and hypersecretion.

12. Patients taking medications for treatment for ulcers on a regular basis should be instructed not to stop medications _abruptly_ to prevent rebound hypersecretion of gastric acid.

13. The health care practitioner should emphasize to the patient and family about delayed release proton pump inhibitors capsules not to chew or crush these medications but they can be _sprinkled_ on food and swallowed immediately with water.

14. Mesalamine and sulfasalazine, two medications that have chemical structures similar to aspirin, exhibit _anti_ - _unflammatory_ activity in the gastrointestinal tract.

15. The salicylates mesalamine and sulfasalazine are used in the management of _Crohn's_ disease and _ulcerative_ colitis.

16. Salicylates bypass the stomach and upper intestines and demonstrate anti-inflammatory activity when reaching the ileum and the _colon_.

82

17. Oral _____steroid_____ have an anti-inflammatory effect after being absorbed into the system and do not require direct contact with inflamed intestinal tissue to be effective.

18. The drugs diphenoxlate with atropine (Lomotil) and loperamide (Imodium) act by slowing intestinal _____motility_____ resulting in an antidiarrheal effect.

19. Antidiarrheals such as Lomotil and Imodium are _____contraindicated_____ in patients with diarrhea caused by infection or food poisoning, in patients with ulcerative colitis, or colitis associated with broad-spectrum antibiotics.

20. Lactinex, an acid-producing bacterium in culture, can be used to treat _____simple_____ diarrhea caused by infection, antibiotics, irritable bowel, colostomy, or amebiasis.

21. The antiflatulent medication _____simethicone_____ is used for symptomatic relief of gastric bloating and postoperative gas pains by breaking up gas bubbles in the gastrointestinal tract.

22. The laxatives of choice for laxative-dependent patients and for older adults are in the category _____bulk_____ _____forming_____ .

23. Patients should be cautioned to avoid use of stool softeners for more than one _____week_____ without medical supervision and to be sure the laxative does not contain any cathartics.

24. The use of mineral oil as a laxative is contraindicated in children under the age of _____five_____ and those patients who are bedridden or debilitated.

25. There is a danger of a ruptured appendix with the use of _____stimulant_____ laxatives.

26. Lactulose is an _____osmotic_____ laxative that draws water from the tissues into the feces and reflexively stimulates evacuation.

27. Medications used in the treatment and/or prevention of nausea, vomiting, or motion sickness are called _____antiemetic_____

28. The antihistamine _____Meclazine_____ (Antivert) is used in the prevention and treatment of nausea, vomiting, and vertigo associated with motion sickness and Meniere's disease.

29. Phenergan can be given IM or IV but should never be given _____subcu_____ .

30. Geriatric patients and those who are debilitated or emaciated will most likely require a _____ dosage of an antiemetic.

31. The serotonin receptor antagonists ondansetron (Zofran) and dolasetron (Anzemet) are used for prevention and treatment of postoperative nausea and vomiting and for patients undergoing _____ .

32. The dopamine-receptor antagonist _____metoclopramide_____ (Reglan) is used on a short-term basis for GI motility disorder, especially gastric _____distress_____ .

Multiple Choice

Circle the letter that best answers the question.

1. Constipation can be a side effect of which of these antacids?

    A. Magnesium antacids
    B. Sodium phosphate
    C. Magnesium citrate and Maalox
    D. Aluminum or calcium carbonate

2. The health care practitioner administering Mylanta, Gelusil, and Maalox explains that these antacids are made from a combination of:

    A. Pepcid and Tagamet.
    B. Aluminum and magnesium.
    C. Calcium carbonate and Cytotec.
    D. Sodium bicarbonate and Nexium.

3. Osteoporosis can be a side effect of frequent use of which of these antacids?

   A. Aluminum
   B. Magnesium
   C. Calcium carbonate
   D. Prilosec

4. When a patient uses over-the-counter antacids for over two weeks without medical supervision, there is a danger of:

   A. Mild gynecomastia.
   B. Mental confusion.
   C. Ineffective liver metabolism.
   D. Masking the symptoms of GI bleeding or GI malignancy.

5. Which antiulcer agent administered on an empty stomach reacts with hydrochloric acid in the stomach to form a paste that adheres to the mucosa providing protection to the ulcer from irritation?

   A. Cytotec.
   B. Tagamet.
   C. Carafate.
   D. Pepcid.

6. Which of these antiulcer agents reduces gastric acid secretion by acting as an H_2 blocker?

   A. Rantidine.
   B. Sucralfate.
   C. Aciphex.
   D. Cytotec.

7. Most peptic ulcer disease is related to which of these conditions?

   A. Infection with *Helicobacter pylori*.
   B. Excessive secretion of sodium bicarbonate.
   C. Gastroesophageal reflux disease.
   D. Esophogitis.

8. Medications that reduce gastric juices and are taken on a regular basis for extended periods can deplete the intrinsic factor necessary for absorption of vitamin

   A. A
   B. C
   C. B_6
   D. B_{12}

9. Spontaneous abortion, dangerous uterine bleeding, and/or maternal or fetal death are all possible side effects of which of the following medications?

   A. Prilosec
   B. Cytotec
   C. Protonix
   D. Dicyclomine

10. Misoprostol (Cytotec) and magnesium-type antacids should not be given to patients because of the potential of exacerbating which of the following adverse effects?

    A. Menstrual irregularities
    B. Headache
    C. Dizziness
    D. Diarrhea

11. Prilosec, Aciphex, Protonix, and Nexium, used in the short-term treatment of gastroesophageal reflux disease, gastric or duodenal ulcers, and erosive esophagitis, are classified in which category?

    A. Antispasmodics/anticholinergics
    B. H₂-receptor antagonists
    C. Proton pump inhibitors
    D. Synthetic analogs

12. Which of these medications should be taken with food in order to minimize diarrhea?

    A. Carafate
    B. Cytotec
    C. Simethicone
    D. Dicyclomine

13. Patients suffering from infection with *Helicobacter pylori* have been successfully treated with multiple drug regimens over a 14-day period such as Prevpac, which contains:

    A. Amoxicillin, clarithromycin, and Prevacid.
    B. Clarithromycin, hyoscyamine, and Tagamet.
    C. Amoxicillin, Carafate, and Nexium.
    D. Dicylomine, Lomotil, and Pepcid.

14. Dicylomine is used as an adjunct therapy in the management of peptic ulcer disease and hypermotility disorders in the gastrointestinal and lower urinary tracts and works by:

    A. Reducing the production and secretion of acid.
    B. Decreasing the smooth muscle tone and motility.
    C. Preventing complications and aid in healing.
    D. Protecting the stomach and bladder lining from irritation.

15. Older adults who take dicyclomine may develop which of these side effects?

    A. Diarrhea and headache.
    B. Bradycardia and increased secretions from mucous membranes.
    C. Tachycardia and confusion.
    D. Vomiting and diarrhea.

16. Which proton pump inhibitors can be administered without regard to food?

    A. Nexium
    B. Prilosec
    C. Protonix
    D. Prevacid

17. Which of these medications have chemical structures similar to aspirin and exhibit anti-inflammatory activity in the gastrointestinal tract?

    A. Mesalamine and sulfasalazine.
    B. Prednisone and prednisolone.
    C. Lomotil and Imodium.
    D. Simethicone and Lactinex.

18. Interactions with the salicylate sulfasalazine include which of the following?

    A. Hyperglycemia with oral diabetic agents
    B. Decreased bone marrow suppression with methotrexate
    C. Increased risk of hemorrhage with warfarin
    D. Increased efficacy with cyclosporine

19. Which oral steroids are used to treat moderate-to-severe forms of inflammatory bowel disease that are poorly controlled with salicylates?

    A. Mesalamine and sulfasalazine.
    B. Prednisone and prednisolone.
    C. Lomotil and Imodium.
    D. Simethicone and Lactinex.

20. The acid-producing bacterium in culture, *Lactobacillus*, helps reestablish normal intestinal flora when given orally for simple diarrhea; however, it is contraindicated in patients with:

    A. Irritable bowel disease.
    B. Amebiasis.
    C. Prosthetic heart valves.
    D. Gastritis.

21. Psyllium, cellulose derivatives, polycarbophil, malt soup extract, and bran are all examples of which type of laxatives?

    A. Hyperosmotic.
    B. Stimulant.
    C. Saline.
    D. Bulk-forming.

22. Which information should the patient receiving a bulk-forming laxative receive from the health care practitioner?

    A. Dissolve all of the bulk-forming laxative completely in one full glass of liquid and follow with another glass of fluid to prevent obstruction.
    B. They should be stopped acute abdominal pain develops.
    C. They take at least one week to be effective.
    D. They can be administered every four hours.

23. Which of these laxatives has an onset of action in six to eight hours?

    A. Docusate
    B. Psyllium
    C. Mineral oil
    D. Glycerin suppository

24. Which of these medications is categorized as a saline laxative and should not be used on a long-term basis?

    A. Castor oil
    B. Mineral oil
    C. Citrate of magnesia
    D. Miralax

25. Which of these medications is categorized as a stimulant laxative with long-term resulting in loss of normal bowel function and/or laxative dependence?

    A. Miralax
    B. Bisacodyl
    C. Psyllium
    D. Docusate

26. Which of these medications are related to the phenothiazines or antihistamines and are ordered to control nausea and vomiting?

    A. Phenergan, Compazine, and Tigan
    B. Reglan, Cystospaz, and Aciphex
    C. Mylicon and Amphogel
    D. Cytotec and meclizine

27. Which of these drugs are used for prophylaxis of motion sickness?

    A. Dramamine and scopolamine
    B. Phenergan and Tigan
    C. Compazine and Aciphex
    D. Dulcolax and lactulose

28. Which of these medications is an antihistamine and is used for the treatment of vertigo associated with motion sickness?

    A. Dimenhydrinate (Dramamine)
    B. Meclizine (Antivert)
    C. Ondansetron (Zofran)
    D. Metoclopramide (Reglan)

29. Which of these medications is a dopamine-receptor antagonist, an antiemetic, and a stimulant of upper GI motility accelerating gastric emptying and intestinal transit?

    A. Dimenhydrinate (Dramamine)
    B. Meclizine (Antivert)
    C. Ondansetron (Zofran)
    D. Metoclopramide (Reglan)

30. Scopolamine in the form of the transdermal patch Transderm–Scop is ordered by the physician to prevent:

    A. Diarrhea.
    B. Abdominal bloating.
    C. Motion sickness.
    D. Smooth muscle spasms in the GI tract.

Matching A

Match the drug in Column A with the category in Column B. Note that the choices in Column B can be used more than once.

COLUMN A	COLUMN B
_____ 1. Bentyl	A. Proton pump inhibitors
_____ 2. Mylicon	B. H_2-blockers
_____ 3. Maalox	C. Antiflatulent
_____ 4. Tums	D. Antidiarrheal agent
_____ 5. Lomotil	E. Salicylates
_____ 6. Bacid	F. Antispasmodic/anticholinergic
_____ 7. AlternaGel	G. Aluminum antacids
_____ 8. Aciphex	H. Calcium carbonate antacids
_____ 9. Zantac	I. Aluminum magnesium combination antacids
_____ 10. Carafate	J. Gastric mucosal agents
_____ 11. Azulfidine	K. Probiotic
_____ 12. Imodium	
_____ 13. Cytotec	
_____ 14. Zantac 75	
_____ 15. Prilosec OTC	
_____ 16. Pepcid	

Matching B

Match the trade name of the drug in Column A with its generic name in Column B.

COLUMN A	COLUMN B
_____ 1. Tagamet	A. Rabeprazole
_____ 2. Pepcid	B. Mesalimine
_____ 3. Zantac	C. Omeprazole
_____ 4. Nexium	D. Misoprostol
_____ 5. Prevacid	E. Cimetidine
_____ 6. Prilosec OTC	F. Sucralfate
_____ 7. Protonix	G. Famotidine
_____ 8. Aciphex	H. Sulfasalazine
_____ 9. Mylicon	I. Loperamide
_____ 10. Bentyl	J. Dicylomine
_____ 11. Lomotil	K. Ranitidine
_____ 12. Imodium	L. Esomeprazole
_____ 13. Carafate	M. Lansoprazole
_____ 14. Cytotec	N. Pantoprazole
_____ 15. Azulfidine	O. Simethicone
_____ 16. Rowasa	P. Diphenoxylate with atropine

Matching C

Match the trade name of the drug in Column A with the category of the drug in Column B. Note that the choices in Column B can be used more than once.

COLUMN A	COLUMN B
_____ 1. Sorbitol	A. Bulk-forming laxative
_____ 2. Dramamine	B. Stool softener
_____ 3. Zofran	C. Stimulant laxative
_____ 4. Dulcolax	D. Saline laxative
_____ 5. Phenergan	E. Osmotic laxative
_____ 6. Antivert	F. Dopamine-receptor antagonist, antiemetic
_____ 7. Miralax	G. Phenothiazine antiemetic
_____ 8. Reglan	H. Prophylaxis of motion sickness, antiemetic
_____ 9. Milk of Magnesia	I. Antihistamine, treatment of vertigo, antiemetic
_____ 10. Senokot	J. Preoperative or chemotherapy antiemetic
_____ 11. Colace	
_____ 12. Metamucil	

True or False

Circle T for true or F for false after reading each of the following statements.

1. T   F   Antacids are given for indigestion and heartburn and can only be purchased at the pharmacy with a note from a physician.

2. T   F   Antacids should be taken at least 2 hours before or 2 hours after other medications to avoid altering the effectiveness of the other medications.

3. T   F   The effectiveness of thyroid hormones may be decreased when taken with antacids.

4. T   F   Patients taking medications for the management of esophageal reflux should also be taught to avoid constrictive clothing, to eat smaller meals, and to avoid lying flat immediately after meals.

5. T   F   Patients taking the H_2-blocker Pepcid have a greater chance of having drug interactions than those taking the H_2-blockers Tagamet or Zantac.

6. T   F   Misoprostol (Cytotec) is an example of a proton pump inhibitor.

7. T   F   The drug of choice for a woman who is pregnant and has a gastric ulcer is misoprostol (Cytotec).

8. T   F   Long-term regular use of agents that reduce gastric acid in older adult patients can have the outcome of vitamin B_{12} deficiency.

9. T   F   Sucralfate (Carafate) should be administered after the client eats breakfast.

10. T   F   GI anticholinergics such as dicyclomine work by decreasing smooth muscle, resulting in decreased motility of the GI tract.

11. T   F   Stool softeners are the laxative of choice for pregnant or nursing women and for children having hard, dry stools.

12. T   F   Bismuth subsalicylate (Kaopectate) has anti-infective and antisecretory properties.

13. T   F   The salicylate sulfasalazine interacts with oral diabetic agents, resulting in hypoglycemia.

14. T   F   Prednisone, prednisolone, and hydrocortisone enemas are glucocorticoids used to treat difficult forms of inflammatory bowel disease in patients who are unsuccessfully controlled with salicylates.

15. T   F   Lactinex should not be taken by patients who are sensitive to milk products.

16. T   F   The antiflatulent simethicone is prescribed for patients with gastric bloating and those suffering from postoperative gas pains to break up gas bubbles in the GI tract.

17. T   F   Patients should be taught to take bulk-forming laxatives with at least 2 ounces of water.

18. T   F   Stool softeners are contraindicated in patients with acute abdominal pain.

19. T   F   Mineral oil can be administered rectally as an oil-retention enema.

20. T   F   Mineral oil should be used with stool softeners to improve bowel evacuation.

Case Study

Philip Kitchen, a 55-year-old man, was admitted for observation to an outpatient clinic following an episode of severe chest pain. His symptoms include substernal chest pain, reflux heartburn, feeling of fullness, sore throat, and hoarseness. It has been determined that Mr. Kitchen has a hiatal hernia, gastric ulcer, and GERD. Mr. Kitchen will need instructions about his new regime, which includes taking Maalox, simethicone, and Prevacid, and dietary and lifestyle management.

1. As the health care provider instructing Mr. Kitchen about his medication, it is important to

   A. Explain the significant complications of not taking his medications correctly.
   B. Teach him and his wife about the correct administration techniques and side effects of his medications.
   C. Show him the X-rays so that he can see how he was diagnosed.
   D. Inform him and his wife about his medical diagnosis and prognosis.

2. The health care practitioner should teach Mr. Kitchen that Prevacid is a

   A. Aluminum-magnesium combination antacid that should be taken 2 hours before or after meals and other medications
   B. Calcium carbonate plus simethicone tablet that should be taken immediately after meals without regard to other medications
   C. Antispasmodic/anticholinergic preparation that should be taken at least 30 minutes before meals
   D. Proton pump inhibitor that should be administered before breakfast and at bedtime

3. The health care practitioner should teach Mr. Kitchen that Maalox should be taken:

   A. 2 hours before or after meals and other medications
   B. immediately after meals without regard to other medications
   C. at least 30 minutes before meals
   D. before breakfast and at bedtime

4. The health care practitioner should teach Mr. Kitchen his treatment regimen should also include

   A. Cigarette smoking to decrease gastric acidity
   B. Increase aerobic exercise
   C. Identify and reduce stress factors
   D. Stop medications if symptoms are not alleviated

CHAPTER 17

Anti-Infective Drugs

Fill-in-the-Blank

Fill in the blank for each of the following statements.

1. The key to treatment of infections is the identification of the _____ organism that is accomplished by a culture and sensitivity test based on symptoms.

2. Culture and sensitivity tests should always be completed _____ beginning anti-infective medication.

3. According to the U.S. Centers for Disease Control and Prevention (CDC), more than 70% of bacteria that cause _____ (hospital-acquired) infections are resistant to at least one of the drugs most commonly used to treat those infections.

4. One of the most effective strategies at combating antimicrobial resistance is strict adherence to preventive measures such as routine _____ .

5. Antimicrobial resistance is increasing in prevalence and also across all _____ of antibiotics.

6. An example of an organism resistant to most antibiotics is MRSA, which stands for methicillin-resistant _____ _____ .

7. Infections such as bacteremia, endocarditis, or urinary tract infections caused by _____ _____ enterococci (VRE) are extremely difficult to treat.

8. The physician must determine the status of hepatic and _____ function prior to the selection of the anti-infective drug.

9. Lower dosages or alternate drugs might be indicated in _____ and older adults because some anti-infectives are more toxic in patients in these age groups.

10. Anti-infectives such as streptomycin and _____ , if administered during pregnancy, can cross the placenta and cause damage to the developing fetus.

11. Combination medications are used to treat tuberculosis to decrease the risk of developing _____ to a single medication.

12. If a patient has an adverse reaction of direct toxicity after receiving an anti-infective, the health care practitioner's responsibility is to assess the patient's physical condition and laboratory reports and potentially _____ the medication.

13. Because cephalosporins are semisynthetic antibiotic derivatives produced by a fungus and are related to the penicillins, patients allergic to _____ who are taking a cephalosporin must be observed very closely for an allergic reaction.

14. The CDC recommends that in the last quarter of each year, flu vaccine be administered to all older adults, immune compromised patients, patients with serious medical conditions and all _____ _____ _____ who have contact with patients at-risk.

15. The health care practitioner has a responsibility to stress the importance of _____ influenza vaccine to high-risk patients to prevent serious, possibly fatal, complications from contracting virulent forms of influenza.

16. Every health care practitioner should teach patients receiving gentamycin and other _____ to report any problems with urinary output or hearing because of the serious side effects of nephrotoxicity and/or ototoxicity.

17. A culture and sensitivity test is may be helpful to determine which cephalosporin is appropriate depending on the _____ recovered.

18. In patients taking a calcium channel blocker such as diltiazem, the macrolide _____ is contraindicated because the combination can cause abnormal, potentially fatal, cardiac arrhythmias.

19. Patients taking antibiotics may include _____ or buttermilk in their diets as they may help regulate intestinal flora and reduce the incidence of diarrhea.

20. For patients exposed to active tuberculosis or who have a significantly positive PPD skin test, even though they are asymptomatic, recommended treatment consists of daily administration of _____ (INH) for six to twelve months to prevent development of active disease.

21. Clindamycin is frequently prescribed for the treatment of *Pneumocysti jirovecii* pneumonia associated with _____ , serious respiratory tract infections, septicemia, osteomylitis, and serious infections of the female pelvis caused by susceptible bacteria.

22. Metronidazole (Flagyl) is a synthetic antibacterial and antiprotozoal agent which is effective against _____ , amebiasis, and giardiasis and useful in treatment of Crohn's disease and antibiotic-related diarrhea.

23. The primary approach to treatment of human immunodeficiency virus (HIV) infection is _____ of the virus at different stages in its reproduction.

24. Eradication of human immunodeficiency virus infection cannot be achieved with currently available _____ regimens.

25. Treatment of HIV-infected patients is complex due to the availability of _____ antiretroviral agents and the rapid growth of new information.

26. Kaposi's sarcoma and toxoplasmosis are examples of _____ infections that occur because the immune system is compromised.

27. Antiviral drugs called _____ are sometimes used in the palliative treatment of AIDS-related Kaposi's sarcoma in adults who are otherwise asymptomatic and not severely immuno-compromised.

28. For prevention of opportunistic infections in HIV-infected children and in adults with CD41T-cell counts less than 200, _____ aerosolized oral inhalation can be used.

29. The health care worker should instruct patients taking a sulfonamide that _____ reactions, which can be fatal, may occur as a possible side effects.

30. Patients taking the urinary anti-infective nitrofurantoin (Furadantin and Macrodantin) should be told that their urine might turn _____ in color and must be taken for a defined time period to be effective.

Multiple Choice

Circle the letter that best answers the question.

1. Pending the results of a culture and sensitivity (C & S) and the patient's history, the physician may order which of these?

   A. Streptomycin
   B. Vancomycin
   C. Tamiflu
   D. An empiric anti-infective regimen

2. Which of these is an example of an indirect toxic reaction to an anti-infective?

   A. Blood dyscrasias, hepatotoxicity, ototoxicity, and nephrotoxicity
   B. Occurrence of hives and/or mild fever
   C. Chest constriction, dyspnea, shock, or collapse occurring suddenly
   D. Inflamed tongue, stomatitis, vaginal yeast infection, and/or diarrhea

3. The most up-to-date information regarding vaccines, immunizations recommendations and requirements can be obtained by contacting the:

   A. U.S. Health and Human Services Department.
   B. U.S. Centers for Disease Control and Prevention.
   C. Local health department.
   D. Patient's family physician.

4. Aminoglycosides are used to treat which of these gram-negative bacterial infections?

   A. Escherichia coli
   B. Staphylococcus aureus
   C. Helicobacter pylori
   D. Trichomonas vaginalis

5. Which of these aminoglycosides are used to combat serious infections?

   A. Vibramycin and tetracycline
   B. Zithromax and clarithromycin
   C. Vancomycin and Zyvox
   D. Gentamycin and amikacin

6. Which of these anti-infectives might be a component of the initial regimen for treatment of tuberculosis?

   A. Kanamycin
   B. Neomycin
   C. Streptomycin
   D. Tobramycin

7. For a patient receiving aminoglycosides serum levels (peak and trough) are drawn. Which description of drawing peak and trough serum levels is correct?

   A. Peak levels are drawn 30 minutes before the infusion or IM injection is administered and trough levels drawn 1 hour after medication is completed.
   B. Trough level is drawn 30 minutes before the medication is administered and peak level should be drawn 1 hour after medication is completed.
   C. Peak level should be drawn 1 hour after the start of the infusion or IM injection; trough level will be drawn 30 minutes before the next dose.
   D. Peak level will be drawn 30 minutes before the medication is administered and trough level should be drawn 1 hour after medication is completed.

8. An increased risk of nephrotoxicity occurs with cephalosporins when are administered with:

   A. Loop diuretics and aminoglycosides.
   B. Tetracycline and aspirin.
   C. Macrolides and loop diuretics.
   D. Aspirin and penicillins.

9. Which of these antibiotics is used in patients allergic to penicillin and preferred in patients with renal disease, pregnant women, and small infants?

   A. Streptomycin
   B. Cefoxitin
   C. Erythromycin
   D. Gentamycin

10. Which of these antibiotics is considered the drug of choice for treatment of syphilis and for prophylactic use in preventing recurrences of rheumatic fever?

    A. Cefadroxil
    B. Paromomycin
    C. Penicillin
    D. Tetracycline

11. The antibiotic piperacillin used to treat organisms such as *Pseudomonas* and is classified as a

    A. Extended-spectrum semisynthetic penicillin.
    B. Penicillin/beta-lactamase inhibitor combination.
    C. Natural penicillin.
    D. Penicillin-resistant penicillin.

12. Which anti-infective is effective against protozoa such as *Trichomonas vaginalis* and against amebiasis and giardiasis?

    A. Metronidazole (Flagyl)
    B. Clindamycin (Cleocin)
    C. Linezolid (Zyvox)
    D. Nystatin

13. Patients taking antibiotics from which of the following categories should be taught to avoid strenuous exercise both during and several weeks after therapy because of the potential side effect of cartilage or tendon damage?

    A. Penicillins
    B. Cephalosporins
    C. Macrolides
    D. Quinolones

14. Which anti-infective is used predominantly in the treatment of herpes simplex, herpes zoster, and varicella zoster infections?

    A. Clindamycin
    B. Flagyl
    C. Acyclovir
    D. Vancomycin

15. Which of these antifungal agents is widely prescribed because it is effective against many fungal pathogens without serious toxicity?

    A. Clindamycin
    B. Flagyl
    C. Acyclovir
    D. Vancomycin

16. Which antibiotic structurally unrelated to other available antibiotics is the drug of choice in the treatment of MRSA?

    A. Clindamycin
    B. Flagyl
    C. Acyclovir
    D. Vancomycin

17. Which of these antibiotics is the newest agent approved to target both MRSA and is also effective in treating diabetic foot infections?

    A. Amantadine
    B. Linezolid
    C. Vancomycin
    D. Arimidex

18. In high-risk patients, which of these antiviral agents is used for the prophylaxis and symptomatic treatment of respiratory infections caused by influenza A virus strains, yet has no effect on influenza B or other viruses?

    A. Amantadine
    B. Linezolid
    C. Oseltamivir
    D. Ribavirin

19. The initial treatment for active tuberculosis includes:

    A. INH given once daily for 2 months.
    B. Rifampin and IM streptomycin until culture conversion.
    C. A combination of ethambutol and streptomycin for 2 months, then INH and ethambutol for 3 months.
    D. A combination of INH, rifampin, pyrazinamide and either ethambutol or IM streptomycin until culture conversion and 3 months beyond.

20. Which vitamin is given with INH to reduce the risk of central nervous system effects and peripheral neuropathy?

    A. Vitamin A
    B. Vitamin B_6
    C. Vitamin B_{12}
    D. Vitamin C

21. Which dosage is suggested for children taking INH and rifampin?

    A. 10 mg/kg of INH and 15 mg/kg of rifampin
    B. 300 mg of INH and 2 g of rifampin
    C. 25–30 mg/kg INH and 25 mg/kg of rifampin
    D. 1,600 mg of INH and 600 of rifampin

22. Which of these medications used to treat HIV/AIDS infections is classified as a non-nucleoside reverse transcriptase inhibitor (NNRTI)?

    A. Ritonavir (Norvir)
    B. Enfuvirtide (Fuzeon)
    C. Nevirapine (Viramune)
    D. Abacavir (Ziagen)

23. The treatment of HIV infection consists of using highly active antiretroviral therapy (HAART). What is the usual therapeutic regimen for these agents?

    A. Only one antiretroviral agent can be used.
    B. One antiretroviral agent is used to begin with, then 2 agents are added after two weeks.
    C. Two antiretroviral agents are administered in combination for 2 weeks and then one agent.
    D. Combination of three or more antiretroviral agents is used.

24. The combination sulfonamides (Bactrim, Septra) are currently used alone or in combination for treatment of which of these clinical situations?

    A. acute complicated UTIs
    B. peptic ulcer disease
    C. hepatitis
    D. leukemia

25. Of the following, which is used most commonly for initial or urinary tract infections caused by susceptible organisms?

    A. Nitrofurantoin
    B. Phenazopyridine
    C. Trimethoprim
    D. Clindamycin

Matching A

Match the anti-infective agent in Column A with the category in Column B. Note that the choices in Column B can be used more than once.

COLUMN A	COLUMN B
_____ 1. Rifampin	A. Aminoglycosides
_____ 2. Nystatin	B. Cephalosporins
_____ 3. Doxycycline	C. Macrolides
_____ 4. Ethambutol	D. Penicillins
_____ 5. Amphotericin B	E. Tetracyclines
_____ 6. Ciprofloxacin	F. Antifungals
_____ 7. Isoniazid	G. Quinolones
_____ 8. Tobramycin	H. Antituberculosis
_____ 9. Erythromycin	
_____ 10. Amoxicillin	
_____ 11. Cefaclor	
_____ 12. Levofloxacin	
_____ 13. Ceftriaxone	

Matching B

Match the key medication in Column A with the description in Column B.

COLUMN A	COLUMN B
_____ 1. Acyclovir	A. Antiviral used in the treatment of parkinsonian syndrome and prophylaxis and symptomatic relief of influenza A virus strains
_____ 2. Metronidazole (Flagyl)	B. Side effects include myelosuppression lactic, acidosis, and pseudomembranous colitis; interacts with antidepressants, beta blockers, radiographic contrast media, and foods and beverages high in tyramine
_____ 3. Ribavirin	C. Side effects include ototoxicity, nephrotoxicity, anaphylaxis, and vascular collapse (hypersensitivity reactions reported in 5%–10% of patients)
_____ 4. Linezolid (Zyvox)	D. Used via nasal and oral inhalation for the treatment of children with severe lower respiratory tract infections
_____ 5. Oseltamivir (Tamiflu)	E. Initial oral treatment is most effective treatment for herpes to relieve pain and speed healing of lesions, although parenteral treatment is recommended in children and immuno-compromised patients
_____ 6. Vancomycin	F. Oral neuraminidase inhibitor indicated for the treatment of uncomplicated acute illness due to influenza A and B
_____ 7. Zanamivir (Relenza)	G. One of the most effective drugs available against anaerobic bacterial infections and is a highly lethal antimicrobial (resistance is almost nonexistent)
_____ 8. Amantadine	H. A neuraminidase inhibitor given via inhalation with its main side effect being airway irritation and bronchospasm (especially in patients with COPD and asthma)
_____ 9. Saquinavir (Fortovase)	I. An antiretroviral protease inhibitor used in the treatment of human immunodeficiency virus and AIDS infections

True or False

Circle T for true or F for false after reading each of the following statements.

1. T F Organisms can build up resistance to anti-infective agents, forcing these drugs to lose their effectiveness because of frequent usage.

2. T F Antibiotics are effective against viruses such as the ones that cause the common cold.

3. T F Vaccines and immunizations administered to children and adults are the same today as they were 10 years ago.

4. T F Many infections caused by gram-negative bacteria are treated with aminoglycosides in combination with other antibiotics.

5. T F Patients being treated with aminoglycosides should be taught to carefully observe their intake and urinary output.

6. T F Cephalosporins are semisynthetic antibiotic derivatives produced by a fungus.

7. T F Aminoglycosides are usually administered parenterally, IV or IM, because of poor absorption from the GI tract.

8. T F Patients receiving cephalosporins should be instructed to avoid alcohol in order to avoid the potential of flushing, tachycardia, and possible shock.

9. T F Patients taking theophylline should not take quinolones because they can potentiate serious or fatal CNS effects, cardiac arrest, or respiratory failure.

10. T F Metronidazole (Flagyl) is the drug of choice for children's infections.

11. T F Adverse side effects of clindamycin include rash, pruritus, fever, and, occasionally, anaphylaxis.

12. T F Vancomycin is the drug of choice for methicillin-resistant *Staphylococcus aureus* (MRSA).

13. T F Vancomycin should not be used for prophylaxis and must be restricted to cases in which it is necessary.

14. T F Although vancomycin is poorly absorbed after oral administration, sometimes it is given orally to treat GI infections such as pseudomembranous colitis due to overgrowth of *C. difficile*.

15. T F Famciclovir has a similar spectrum of activity to acyclovir; however, the dosage is less frequent and it has a longer duration of action.

16. T F The antiviral agent amantadine is recommended as a substitute for the influenza vaccination.

17. T F The culture and sensitivity test will identify the specific anti-infective medication that will best eradicate the causative organism.

18. T F Hyperglycemia, new-onset diabetes mellitus, diabetic ketoacidosis, and exacerbation of existing diabetes are side effects of the antiretroviral protease inhibitors.

19. T F Patients receiving treatment for HIV infection with the combination antiretrovirals (HAART) have a reduced risk of transmission of HIV to others through sexual contact or blood contamination.

20. T F Health care practitioners who administer pentamidine inhalation therapy to HIV-infected patients should be aware of the possibility of exposure to tuberculosis in cough-inducing procedures.

21. T F Urinary anti-infectives are usually bacteriostatic instead of bactericidal in action.

22. T F Patients should be taught that their secretions such as urine and sweat would turn a red-orange color when taking rifampin.

Case Study

Sandy Mode, a 45-year-old homeless man, has been diagnosed with active tuberculosis. He is asked to come to the clinic once a week until his medications, a combination of INH, rifampin, pyrazinamide, and ethambutol, can be regulated.

1. The health care practitioner at the clinic recognizes that this patient's medications are categorized as which type of agents?

    A. Antiviral
    B. Antiretroviral
    C. Antifungal
    D. Antituberculosis

2. The health care practitioner's should teach the patient about what potential side effects of INH?

    A. Visual problems (optic neuritis)
    B. Gout—increased uric acid
    C. Weakness or numbness in the extremities
    D. Problems with urination

3. The health care practitioner should teach the patient that when taking rifampin:

    A. If flulike symptoms occur, stop medication.
    B. Body fluids will be red-orange colored.
    C. Drinking alcohol is acceptable.
    D. Jaundice may occur.

4. What effects will the health care practitioner teach the patient about ethambutol?

    A. Drinking alcohol is acceptable.
    B. Body secretions will turn blue.
    C. Report any visual problems (optic neuritis).
    D. Urinary output will be reduced.

5. The health care practitioner should explain to the patient that some combinations of the prescribed medications must be taken for how many months?

    A. 2
    B. 5
    C. 4
    D. 6

CHAPTER 18

Eye Medications

Fill-in-the-Blank

Fill in the blank for each of the following statements.

1. When treating a superficial eye infection with a topical ophthalmc ointment, improvement should be noted within two to _____ days.

2. Eyedrops or eye ointment are correctly instilled into the _____ conjunctival sac to avoid contamination of the tip of the dropper or ointment tube.

3. Prolonged use of anti-infectives for the eye may result in _____ of nonsusceptible organisms, including fungi.

4. The health care practitioner knows that when using more than one ophthalmic product at the same time the more viscous preparation should be administered _____.

5. Herpes simplex, keratitis, or conjunctivitis are treated with _____ ophthalmic preparations.

6. To relieve inflammation of the eye or conjunctiva in allergic reactions, a _____ ophthalmic agent is often used.

7. Prolonged use of ophthalmic corticosteroids should be avoided because of the danger of masking symptoms of _____ or slow the healing process.

8. Nonsteroidal anti-inflammatory drugs (NSAIDs) are used to treat postoperative inflammation following _____ surgery or in other eye conditions with inflammation as an alternative to corticosteroids.

9. Applying gentle pressure on the tear duct at the inner canthus following administration of ophthalmic medications reduces _____ absorption.

10. Glaucoma is an abnormal condition of the eye in which there is increased intraocular pressure due to obstruction of the _____ of aqueous humor.

11. Acute (angle-closure) glaucoma, characterized by sudden onset of pain, blurred vision, and a dilated pupil is considered a _____ _____.

12. Chronic (open-angle) glaucoma develops slowly over a period of years with few symptoms except a gradual loss of _____ vision and possibly blurred vision.

13. Carbonic anhydrase inhibitors reduce the hydrogen and bicarbonate ions, producing a _____ effect.

14. Carbonic anhydrase inhibitors are to be used with caution or _____ in patients with chronic obstructive pulmonary disease, diabetes, and renal disorders.

15. Dorzolamide (Trusopt) is a carbonic anhydrase inhibitor that is applied topically to treat _____ -angle glaucoma.

16. Miotics _____ intraocular pressure by contracting the ciliary muscle, thus increasing the aqueous humor outflow.

17. The miotic _____ is used short term in the treatment of acute angle-closure glaucoma before surgery and to treat chronic open-angle glaucoma.

18. Used for open-angle glaucoma,, the beta-adrenergic blocker _____ may interact with oral beta-blockers to increase chances of hypotension, bradycardia, and heart block.

19. Betaxolol (Betoptic) is a _____ beta-blocker that can be used in patients with bronchospastic pulmonary disease.

20. Epinephrine, an adrenergic, has a _____ effect in patients with open-angle glaucoma but is ineffective as a mydriatic in normal eyes.

21. A pro-drug of epinephrine, dipivefrin (Propine), is ordered more frequently than epinephrine to reduce elevated intraocular pressure in the treatment of chronic open-angle glaucoma because it has _____ side effects.

22. Prostaglandin analogs cause the greatest reduction in intraocular pressure by increasing the _____ of aqueous humor.

23. Patients using prostaglandin analogs should be taught to remove contact lenses prior to administration and leave them out for 15 minutes because this medication contains a _____ that may be absorbed by contact lenses.

24. Patients must be taught to protect their eyes after having a local ophthalmic anesthetic, such as Pontocaine, instilled because of the loss of the _____ reflex.

Multiple Choice

Circle the letter that best answers the question.

1. Which of these medications are examples of ophthalmic antibiotic preparations?

   A. Pilocarpine HCl, dorzolamide, and acetazolamide
   B. Prednisolone, dexamethasone, flurbiprofen
   C. Gentamycin, erythromycin, and polymyxin B
   D. Timolol, brimonidine, and travoprost

2. Which of these medications are examples of corticosteroid anti-inflammatory ophthalmic agents used to relieve inflammation of the conjunctiva?

   A. Flurbiprofen, ketorolac, and acetazolamide
   B. Prednisolone, dexamethasone, fluorometholone
   C. Gentamycin, erythromycin, and polymyxin B
   D. Timolol, brimonidine, and travoprost

3. Which of these categories of antiglaucoma drugs lower intraocular pressure by decreasing the formation of aqueous humor?

   A. Prostaglandin analogs
   B. Beta-Adrenergic blockers
   C. Miotics
   D. Carbonic anhydrase inhibitors

4. Which of these antiglaucoma drugs act to lower intraocular pressure by increasing the aqueous humor outflow?

   A. Beta-adrenergic blockers
   B. Sympathomimetics
   C. Miotics
   D. Carbonic anhydrase inhibitors

5. Dipivefrin, a pro-drug of epinephrine, is included in which category of antiglaucoma drugs?

   A. Prostaglandin analogs
   B. Sympathomimetics
   C. Beta-adrenergic blockers
   D. Carbonic anhydrase inhibitors

6. Latanoprost acts by increasing aqueous outflow and is considered a:

    A. Prostaglandin analog.
    B. Sympathomimetic.
    C. Beta-adrenergic blocker.
    D. Alpha agonist.

7. The effect of which of these medications is decreased when taken with carbonic anhydrase inhibitors?

    A. Quinidine
    B. Amphetamines
    C. Oral antidiabetics
    D. Other diuretics

8. Patients being treated with miotics should be taught to

    A. Close the tear duct after instillation to avoid systemic absorption.
    B. Administer the medication once a day to reduce side effects.
    C. Increase dosage if blurred vision occurs.
    D. Wear special glasses when driving at night.

9. Timolol (Timoptic) acts by decreasing the rate of aqueous humor production and is in which category of ophthalmic medications?

    A. Prostaglandin analog
    B. Sympathomimetic
    C. Beta-adrenergic blocker
    D. Alpha agonist

10. When teaching a patient about administering more than one ophthalmic medication, the health care practitioner should emphasize allowing how much time between doses?

    A. At least 2 minutes
    B. At least 5 minutes
    C. 15 minutes
    D. 30 minutes

11. When a topical ophthalmic beta-blocker is contraindicated, which alternative topical medication is often prescribed?

    A. Brimonidine, a selective alpha agonist
    B. Lantanoprost, a prostaglandin analog
    C. Epinephrine, a sympathomimetic
    D. Pilocarpine, a miotic

12. The mydriatic atropine is the drug of choice for children during:

    A. Detailed eye examinations.
    B. Inspection of the conjunctiva sac for infection.
    C. Checkups for vision screening.
    D. Assessment in order to constrict the pupil.

Matching

Match the medication listed in Column A with the category in Column B. Note that the choices in Column B can be used more than once.

COLUMN A	COLUMN B
_____ 1. Timolol (Timoptic)	A. Mydriatic
_____ 2. Latanoprost (Xalatan)	B. Carbonic anhydrase inhibitor

(*Matching continued on next page*)

COLUMN A **(continued)**	**COLUMN B** **(continued)**

_____ 3. Pilocarpine HCl (Isopto Carpine)   C. Miotics

_____ 4. Travoprost (Travatan)   D. Beta-adrenergic blocker

_____ 5. Cyclopentolate (Cyclogyl)   E. Prostaglandin analogs

_____ 6. Acetazolamide (Diamox)   F. Alpha agonist

_____ 7. Betaxolol   G. Local anesthetic

_____ 8. Brimonidine (Alphagan-P)

_____ 9. Tetracaine (Tetra Visc)

_____ 10. Proparacaine

_____ 11. Atropine (Atropine)

True or False

Circle T for true or F for false after reading each of the following statements.

1. T F Patients should be taught to contact their physician about any signs of sensitivity (burning, itching) after beginning eyedrops or ointment.

2. T F The antiviral ophthalmic solution Viroptic is instilled into the lower conjunctival sac of the infected eye up to nine times a day at 2-hour intervals.

3. T F Pilocarpine is used before an ophthalmic examination in glaucoma patients to dilate the pupil.

4. T F Pilocarpine hydrochloride gel provides increased duration of effectiveness and needs less frequent administration than ophthalmic solutions.

5. T F There are systemic effects with frequent or prolonged use of Pilocarpine especially in children, including hypotension, bradycardia, and bronchospasm.

6. T F Patients treated with beta-adrenergic blockers for glaucoma must be taught the importance of continuous use and not to abruptly discontinue its use.

7. T F Brimonidine, an alpha agonist, decreases the formation of aqueous humor with minimal effects on cardiovascular or pulmonary hemodynamics.

8. T F Slow gradual change in color of the iris is a side effect of prostaglandin analogs.

9. T F After a mydriatic has been administered to a patient, the health care practitioner should recommend wearing dark glasses or staying out of the bright light.

10. T F The patient having minor surgical procedures may have a topical carbonic anhydrase inhibitor instilled to decrease the discomfort of the procedure.

Case Study

Jerry Norton has been taken to the doctor's office because of an eye injury at work. The doctor examines his right eye to determine the severity of the injury.

1. If the doctor instills eyedrops to dilate the pupil these are called:

   A. Local anesthetics.
   B. Miotics.
   C. Sympathomimetics.
   D. Mydriatics.

2. To decrease the pain in Jerry's right eye from the injury or to remove a foreign body, the doctor will probably administer a medication from which of these categories?

   A. Mydriatics
   B. Sympathomimetics
   C. Carbonic anhydrase inhibitors
   D. Local anesthetics

3. After the examination and removal of the piece of steel from Jerry's right eye the doctor instills medication and places an eye patch on the eye. He instructs Jerry to avoid touching or rubbing his eye until the anesthesia is worn off. Which of the following topical medications did he instill into his eye?

   A. Atropine
   B. Brimonidine
   C. Tetra Visc
   D. Timoptic

4. The doctor instructed Jerry to remove the patch the next day and apply one drop of Pred Forte and one drop of gentamycin because they will decrease:

   A. Pupil constriction and discomfort.
   B. Intraocular pressure and to keep the pupil dilated.
   C. Inflammation and prevent infection.
   D. The rate of aqueous humor production and to relieve pain.

5. The health care practitioner instructs Jerry about instilling the eyedrops, explaining that he should instill the first one and wait for what time period before instilling the second?

   A. 2 minutes
   B. 5 minutes
   C. 10 minutes
   D. 15 minutes

6. Jerry should also be taught to apply gentle pressure on the inner canthus following administration of the eyedrops in order to:

   A. Minimize systemic absorption.
   B. Maximize the effectiveness of the drops.
   C. Decrease the risk of infection.
   D. Increase the flow of aqueous humor.

CHAPTER 19

Analgesics, Sedatives, and Hypnotics

Fill-in-the-Blank

Fill in the blank for each of the following statements.

1. The health care practitioner observes a patient in pain and notes that she is crying and holding her head between her hands; this is _____ data.

2. The health care practitioner is aware that some patients experience pain with higher thresholds than others do because of conditioning, _____ background, sensitivity, or physiological factors.

3. Endorphins are _____ analgesics produced as a reaction to pain or intense exercise, such as a "runner's high."

4. The action of full agonist analgesics classified as opioids is similar to that of _____ in altering perception of pain because they have no ceiling to their analgesic effects, that is, medication level where there is no enhanced analgesia.

5. Opioids are listed under the controlled substances schedule in the United States and include both natural opium alkaloids and _____.

6. Pain medications such as Darvon and Darvocet are examples of synthetic opioids that contain the drug _____, which are linked to death from drug overdoses and now require an FDA warning statement emphasizing this risk.

7. The patient who receives an opioid analgesic over a continuous period tend to develop _____ to the drug and will be less responsive to its analgesic effect unless larger doses are administered.

8. Opioids administered consistently may result in the patient's developing physiological _____, leading to withdrawal symptoms when the medication is discontinued abruptly.

9. Sufficient pain control is essential for the terminally ill patient with constant pain and analgesics should be given _____ - _____ _____.

10. The health care practitioner knows that the _____ of opioids with nonopioid medications and adjuvant drugs provides analgesia that is more effective for the terminally ill patient.

11. Terminal pain is best controlled by administering analgesics at regular intervals, with additional as-needed doses for _____ pain.

12. For the patient experiencing _____ pain, the addition of a tricyclic antidepressant or an anticonvulsant to the pain regime will decrease the amount of needed dosage of opioids.

13. Side effects of opioid analgesics can include sedation, dizziness, hypotension, respiratory _____, and bradycardia.

14. Opioid analgesics must be used with extreme _____ in patients with central nervous system depression, head injury, or conditions associated with increased intracranial pressure.

15. The health care practitioner recognizes that _____ is not recommended for routine use due to a metabolite which may accumulate in patients and cause seizures in patients with kidney disease.

16. If opioids are administered with muscle relaxants, antihistamines, psychotropics, or alcohol, the effect of the opioids will be _____.

17. Opioid analgesics are available in various strengths, as concentrated solutions, and in _____ products.

18. An opioid analgesic is usually administered parenterally as a _____ medication.

19. Major side effects of salicylates and other NSAIDS, which occur with prolonged or high dosages, may be silent or may include _____ distress, ulceration, and bleeding.

20. Acetaminophen is an over-the-counter analgesic and is used extensively in the treatment of _____ to moderate pain and fever.

21. Patients taking acetaminophen frequently should be cautioned that alcohol ingestion could lead to potential _____ damage.

22. For the treatment of nerve pain associated with herpes, arthritis, diabetes, cancer, migraine or tension headaches, insomnia, and depression, _____ antidepressants are often prescribed.

23. Tricyclic antidepressants increase available norephinephrine and serotonin, which block pain _____ and thus relieve pain that patients describe as "burning pain."

24. Unlike opioid analgesics in which the therapeutic effect is felt in less than an hour, patients taking tricyclic antidepressants must allow 2–3 _____ to feel full therapeutic effects.

25. For patients in whom oral analgesics may not be a viable option for pain control, _____ is available topically in a patch (Lidoderm).

26. Side effects that may occur when opioid and a tricyclic antidepressant are _____ constipation, hypotension, and sedation.

27. The first-line _____ prescribed for neuropathic pain therapy is babapentin (Neurontin).

28. Serotonin receptor agonists are indicated for the _____ treatment of migraines in adults.

29. The antimigraine agent sumatriptan (Imitrex) has no therapeutic value for the _____ management of migraine headaches.

30. Sedative-hypnotics substances used to promote _____ in smaller doses and promote _____ in larger doses.

31. Antihistamines such as diphenhydramine (Benadryl) have an extended half-life, leading to "morning after" problems when used as _____ _____ in older adults.

32. Sedative-hypnotic medications such as benzodiazepines like temazepam (Restoril) and nonbenzodiazepines like zolpidem (Ambien) are recommended for only _____ _____ use.

Multiple Choice

Circle the letter that best answers the question.

1. Which of the following assessments should the health care practitioner make before administering an analgesic?

   A. Does the patient need to be calmed, soothed, or sedated?
   B. Does the client need medication for sleep?
   C. Is the patient in pain and need medicating?
   D. Has the patient developed a high fever?

2. Which of the following describes subjective pain?

   A. "My arm hurts when I lift something heavy."
   B. BP 158/70, pulse 120, and respirations 30.
   C. Patients grimaces when lifting the suitcase.
   D. Abdominal incision is red and hot to touch.

3. Which of the following is a synthetic opioid?

   A. Demerol
   B. Morphine
   C. Codeine
   D. Tylenol

4. Which of these preparations is a centrally acting synthetic analog of codeine?

   A. meperidine (Demerol)
   B. carbamazepine (Tegretol)
   C. tramadol (Ultram)
   D. hydrocodone (Lorcet)

5. Which of these medications is an opioid antagonist used in the treatment of opioid overdoses and in the delivery room and newborn nursery for opiate-induced respiratory depression?

   A. Tylenol
   B. Meperidine
   C. Atropine
   D. Naloxone

6. Which of these medications is a nonopioid analgesic and anti-inflammatory?

   A. acetylsalicylic acid
   B. acetaminophen
   C. butalbital
   D. caffeine

7. For a more effective analgesic action, which drugs are most frequently combined with opioids or other drugs?

   A. Atropine and Phenergan
   B. Naloxone and naltrexone
   C. Aspirin and acetaminophen
   D. Lidocaine and tegretol

8. High doses or prolonged usage of salicylates or NSAIDs may be discontinued for a period prior to surgery because which of these side effects?

   A. Sodium and water retention
   B. Prolonged bleeding time
   C. Tinnitus
   D. Drowsiness and dizziness

9. Health care practitioners should teach patients taking NSAIDs or salicylates that to minimize GI symptoms, the medications should be taken can be minimized by administering:

   A. On an empty stomach.
   B. 2 hours after eating.
   C. With food or milk.
   D. With a high dose of antacids.

10. NSAIDs and/or salicylates are contraindicated in any patient with which vitamin deficiency?

   A. Vitamin A
   B. Vitamin C
   C. Vitamin D
   D. Vitamin K

11. What is the effect of administering an anticoagulant to a patient who is taking salicylates?

    A. the anticoagulant effect is decreased.
    B. the action of the anticoagulant is potentiated.
    C. the patient's blood will clot faster.
    D. absorption of vitamin is increased.

12. Which of these is one of the most common side effects of salicylates, especially with prolonged use?

    A. tinnitus
    B. dizziness
    C. depression
    D. euphoria

13. Hypersensitivity or overdosage of salicylates, especially in children, may result in which of these conditions?

    A. hepatic dysfunction
    B. gastric distress
    C. coma and respiratory failure
    D. increased urine output

14. While side effects of acetaminophen are rare, with high doses taken too frequently or with an overdose there is a risk of:

    A. Orthostatic hypotension.
    B. Seizure disorder.
    C. Gastric bleeding.
    D. Severe liver toxicity.

15. Which of these statements about Tramadol (Ultram) is true?

    A. It is frequently combined with opioid analgesics when stronger pain relief is required.
    B. It is not classified as a controlled substance.
    C. It has great potential for abuse or respiratory depression.
    D. It is used for treatment of opioid overdosage.

16. Which of these medications are classified as adjuvant analgesics, enhancing analgesic effect with opioids and nonopioids, producing analgesia alone, or reducing the side effects of analgesics?

    A. Hydrocodone and fentanyl.
    B. Meperidine and ramelteon.
    C. Amitriptyline and gabapentin.
    D. Morphine and codeine.

17. Which of the following adjuvant medications is the drug of choice for trigeminal neuralgia?

    A. Amitriptyline
    B. Carbamazepine (Tegretol)
    C. Tramadol (Ultram)
    D. Hydromorphone (Dilaudid)

18. Which of the following adjuvant medications is the drug of choice for post-herpetic neuralgia?

    A. Amitriptyline (Elavil)
    B. Carbamazepine (Tegretol)
    C. Gabapentin (Neurontin)
    D. Tramadol (Ultram)

19. Which of the statements about the treatment of migraine headaches is true?

    A. Serotonin receptor agonists such as Imitrex are effective in the acute treatment of migraines.
    B. It is common for neurovascular headaches to include nausea and/or vomiting and sensitivity to light and/or noise.
    C. Simple analgesics, NSAIDs, and opioid analgesics are usually effective for treating migraines.
    D. Serotonin receptor agonists provide pain relief from migraines.

20. Hypnotic dosage should be gradually reduced because abrupt withdrawal of hypnotics, even after short-term therapy, may result in:

    A. Rebound insomnia.
    B. Maculopapular rash.
    C. Hypotension.
    D. Dehydration.

21. Temazepam (Restoril) and triazolam (Halcion) are used for short term only and are categorized as:

    A. Barbiturates.
    B. Benzodiazepines.
    C. Antimigraine agents.
    D. Local anesthetics.

22. Eletriptan (Relpax) and rizatriptan (Maxalt) are agents from which of these categories?

    A. Barbiturates
    B. Benzodiazepines
    C. Antimigraine
    D. Local anesthetics

Matching A

Match the trade name of the medication listed in Column A with the generic name listed in Column B. Note that the choices in Column B can be used more than once.

COLUMN A	COLUMN B
_____ 1. Stadol	A. Propoxyphene HCl
_____ 2. MS Contin SR	B. Fentanyl citrate
_____ 3. Sublimaze	C. Hydromorphone
_____ 4. Lorcet	D. Propoxyphene HCl with acetaminophen
_____ 5. Dolophine	E. Oxycodone
_____ 6. Demerol	F. Morphine
_____ 7. Lortab	G. Methadone
_____ 8. Duragesic	H. Oxycodone with aspirin
_____ 9. Vicodin	I. Meperidine
_____ 10. Dilaudid	J. Oxycodone with acetaminophen
_____ 11. Darvon	K. Butorphanol
_____ 12. Talwin NX	L. Hydrocodone with acetaminophen
_____ 13. OxyContin	M. Pentazocine
_____ 14. Percodan	
_____ 15. Percocet	
_____ 16. Darvocet	

Matching B

Match the trade name listed in Column A with the generic name listed in Column B. Note that the choices in Column B can be used more than once.

COLUMN A	COLUMN B
_____ 1. Ultram	A. Tramadol with acetaminophen
_____ 2. Anacin	B. Acetylsalicylic acid
_____ 3. Equagesic	C. ASA, acetaminophen, and caffeine
_____ 4. Fioricet	D. Acetaminophen
_____ 5. Excedrin	E. ASA and meprobamate
_____ 6. Panadol	F. Butalbital, caffeine, and acetaminophen
_____ 7. Bufferin	G. Tramadol
_____ 8. Esgic	H. ASA and caffeine
_____ 9. Panadol	
_____ 10. Ascriptin	
_____ 11. Ultracet	
_____ 12. Ecotrin	

True or False

Circle T for true or F for false after reading each of the following statements.

1. T F Sedatives are given to calm, soothe, or produce sedation in patients.

2. T F Salicylate analgesic and anti-inflammatory actions are associated primarily with preventing the formation of prostaglandins.

3. T F The salicylate Tylenol is most commonly used for its analgesic, anti-inflammatory, and antipyretic properties.

4. T F Acetaminophen is ordered for the anti-inflammatory actions it provides.

5. T F Tylenol No. 3 tablets contain 300 mg of acetaminophen and 30 mg of codeine.

6. T F One teaspoon of Tylenol with codeine elixir has 12 mg of codeine and 120 mg of acetaminophen.

7. T F Each Darvocet-N 100 contains 100 mg of acetaminophen and 100 mg of propoxyphene.

8. T F Tinnitus and hearing loss are possible side effects with an overdose of salicylates or other NSAIDs.

9. T F Using Ultram with SSRIs such as Paxil and Zoloft increases seizure risk because serotonin syndrome may develop.

10. T F Serotonin receptor agonists are effective in the prophylactic treatment of migraine headaches.

11. T F Barbiturates are rarely used now, although phenobarbital is still used in treatment of seizure disorders.

12. T F Sedative-hypnotic medications have the potential for psychological and physical dependence.

13. T F Some psychotropic drugs and some antihistamines are used as sedative-hypnotics.

14. T F Benzodiazepines are used for sedation but can lead to dependence and withdrawal symptoms.

15. T F Prior to starting pharmacological treatment for insomnia, patients should be encouraged to use more natural methods, including exercise, warm milk, back rubs, soft music and other calming influences, and avoiding heavy meals near bedtime.

16. T F All sedative-hypnotics are contraindicated for patients who have hypersensitivity.

Case Study

Jim Ginn, 65 years old, is going to have outpatient surgery next week to repair an inguinal hernia repair. As the health care provider at the surgeon's office, you are teaching Jim his about pre-op and post-op medications.

1. What information is important for the health care practitioner to tell the patient?

   A. Regular medications are administered the morning of surgery after breakfast.
   B. Hypnotics are only to be used on a short-term basis.
   C. Antihistamines have an extended half-life, remain in the system longer, and the effects continue for a longer time.
   D. An opioid analgesic will be given as a pre-op medication about 30–60 minutes before the surgery.

2. Which of these medications is likely to be administered preoperatively?

   A. Demerol and atropine
   B. Sublimaze
   C. Diphenhydramine
   D. Imitrex

3. Which post-op pain medication will likely be ordered for Jim during the immediate post-op period?

   A. Atropine
   B. Morphine
   C. Restoril
   D. Phenobarbital

4. If Jim develops respiratory depression from the pain medication, what medication can be administered to reverse the action of the opioid overdose?

   A. Narcan
   B. Hydrocodone
   C. Stadol
   D. Halcion

5. When Jim returns home, he will need a pain medication to relieve moderate-to-severe pain and take it PO. Which of the following may be ordered for this time?

   A. Morphine
   B. Demerol
   C. Percocet
   D. Ambien

6. Jim occasionally takes a hypnotic, zolpidem (Ambien), for sleep. What information should the health care practitioner include when teaching the patient?

   A. Take the analgesic first and wait an hour and then take the hypnotic.
   B. Drink plenty of water with both medications.
   C. Serious potential side effects such as confusion and oversedation may occur.
   D. The hypnotic can be taken in the morning and the analgesic at night to improve the effects.

CHAPTER **20**

Psychotropic Medications, Alcohol, and Drug Abuse

Fill-in-the-Blank

Fill in the blank for each of the following statements.

1. Any substance that acts on the mind is called a _____.

2. Psychotropic medications are drugs that can exert a _____ effect on a person's mental processes, emotions, or behavior.

3. Psychotropic medications are typically ordered concurrently with _____ or professional counseling.

4. One of the most commonly consumed CNS stimulants is _____.

5. CNS stimulants have a high potential for _____ and should be used only under medical supervision for diagnosed medical disorders.

6. Controlled CNS stimulants, including _____ (Adderall) and methylphenidate (Ritalin), are medications ordered for the treatment of attention-deficit hyperactivity disorder or attention-deficit disorder without hyperactivity.

7. Abrupt _____ of CNS stimulants results in depression, headache, irritation, nervousness, and anxiety.

8. Prolonged administration of CNS stimulants in some children can cause _____ of normal weight and/or height patterns.

9. Patients need instruction to take their prescribed CNS stimulant early in the day to reduce _____ as a potential side effect.

10. The tricyclic antidepressants act by the _____ of norepinephrine and serotonin activity by blocking their reuptake presynaptically.

11. The side effects of tricyclics are _____ in action, including dryness of the mouth, constipation, and urinary retention, especially with BPH.

12. MAO inhibitors are rarely used today because of potential serious side effects and numerous _____ with food and drugs.

13. Interactions of the MAO inhibitors with some drugs and foods can cause _____, _____ marked by severe headache, palpitation, sweating, chest pain, possible intracranial hemorrhage, and even death.

14. First-line medications for the treatment of depression are from the _____ category.

15. It is important for patients receiving _____ for a bipolar disorder to be aware of signs of toxicity and have regular serum levels drawn in order to maintain a level of 0.8–1.5 mEq/mL.

111

© 2011 Cengage Learning. All Rights Reserved. May not be scanned, copied or duplicated, or posted to a publicly accessible website, in whole or in part.

16. Because of the development of physical and psychological dependence, sudden withdrawal of benzodiazepines after _____ use may result in seizures, agitation, psychosis, insomnia, and gastric distress.

17. A patient taking buspirone for anxiety will find that the drug has an onset of _____ to _____ weeks for optimum effect, which is a slower onset of action than most anxiolytics.

18. The health care provider administering Versed parenterally will monitor the respiratory status _____ and have equipment for respiratory and cardiovascular support readily available.

19. Typical antipsychotics, such as Thorazine, are classified chemically as phenothiazines and work by _____ dopamine receptors, resulting in unbalanced cholinergic activity.

20. Patients taking typical antipsychotics may develop unwanted _____ side effects and tardive dyskinesia.

21. Extrapyramidal reactions may become permanent and irreversible and include _____ symptoms such as tremors, drooling, and dysphasia.

22. The health care practitioner is aware that extrapyramidal reactions such as tardive dyskinesia (involuntary movements such as tics) and _____ reactions (spasms of the head, neck, or tongue) are adverse reactions to antipsychotic medications.

23. Patients receiving antipsychotics should be assessed for _____ _____ at the start of treatment and at least every 6 months with the Abnormal Involuntary Movement Scale (AIMS) or Dyskinesia Identification System: Condensed User Scale (DISCUS).

24. All patients taking psychotropic drugs should be instructed regarding the potential for psychological and/or _____ dependence with prolonged use and that medications should be taken only in prescribed dosages and under medical supervision.

25. All patients taking psychotropic medications for a prolonged period of time need to be aware of probable _____ reactions when abruptly stopping the medication.

26. Prolonged use of alcohol can cause permanent _____ damage and result in peripheral neuritis, convulsive disorders, Wernicke's syndrome, and Korsakoff's psychosis with mental deterioration, memory loss, and ataxia.

27. Mortality associated with _____ alcohol poisoning alone is uncommon; however, it can be an important factor when mixed with recreational drugs.

28. Fetal alcohol syndrome is a _____ effect of alcohol and more commonly occurs when the mother has consumed four or five drinks per day during pregnancy.

29. Symptoms of chronic abuse of _____ consist of emotional liability, irritability, anorexia, amnesia, neurotoxicity, and tooth decay ("meth mouth").

30. When a person smokes _____, the active ingredient, fat soluble THC, is released, stored in fat cells, and not completely eliminated from the body until 4–6 weeks later.

31. The CNS stimulant _____ is highly addictive and is abused by intranasal application, intravenous injection, or by inhalation.

Multiple Choice

Circle the letter that best answers the question.

1. Which of these statements about tricyclic antidepressants is true?

   A. They are used to provide complete neuropathic pain control
   B. They are administered early morning to increase the patient's alertness
   C. They are more effective than SSRIs in some severe depression
   D. They are used less frequently than the MAO inhibitors

2. MAO inhibitors are typically reserved for use in treating in patients with

   A. cerebrovascular, heart, liver, and renal disease.
   B. refractory or atypical depression.
   C. hypertension.
   D. depression related to smoking cessation.

3. Selective serotonin reuptake inhibitors (SSRIs) selectively block the reabsorption of the neurotransmitter serotonin, and are considered to be the:

   A. First-line drugs for treatment of depression because of fewer side effects and greater safety in cases of overdose and increased patient compliance.
   B. Drugs of choice for treating bipolar disorders.
   C. Activating antidepressants and only useful in cases of severe depression.
   D. Antimanic agents in which blood levels must be monitored every few months to maintain a therapeutic level.

4. Symptomatic relief of depression for patients being treated with SSRIs occurs approximately how long after beginning treatment?

   A. 1 to 4 hours
   B. 1 to 4 days
   C. 1 to 4 weeks
   D. 1 to 4 months

5. One advantage of treatment with SSRIs over other antidepressants is that they:

   A. do not affect sexual function.
   B. can be taken with the MAO inhibitors as needed.
   C. do not have a significant effect on cognition in older adults.
   D. reduce the risk of suicide.

6. Heterocyclic antidepressants such as Buproprion (Wellbutrin) are comparable in efficacy to first-generation tricyclics and are considered to be:

   A. The first choice in treating depression because it produces fewer serious side effects.
   B. An activating antidepressant which can be useful in cases of severe depression.
   C. An antimanic agent in which blood levels must be monitored every few months to maintain a therapeutic level.
   D. The first-line medication for treatment of depression because it selectively blocks the reabsorption of serotonin.

7. One advantage of treatment with heterocyclic antidepressants over other antidepressants is that they:

   A. are less likely to affect sexual function.
   B. can be taken with the MAO inhibitors is needed.
   C. do not have to use caution in patients with cardiac or liver disorders.
   D. pose no risk when administered to suicidal prone patients.

8. Which of these is medications an antimanic agent used to treat bipolar disorders and requires monitoring of serum levels monitored long term to prevent toxicity?

   A. Zoloft
   B. Wellbutrin
   C. Remeron
   D. Lithium

9. Medications in which of these categories are used for short-term treatment of anxiety disorders, some psychosomatic disorders, insomnia, nausea and vomiting, and neurosis while making the patient amenable to psychotherapy?

   A. Antimanics
   B. Anxiolytics
   C. CNS stimulants
   D. SNRIs

10. Which of these medications are classified as benzodiazepines?

    A. Effexor, Strattera, and Symbyax
    B. Tegretol, Depakote, and Desyrel
    C. Xanax, Ativan, Librium, and Tranxene
    D. Paxil, Lexapro, Zoloft, and Prozac

11. Compounds with a long half-life, such as diazepam (Valium), should be avoided in which patients because of the accumulation of the medication?

    A. Older adults and those with liver disease
    B. Children and those with photosensitivity
    C. Anyone who is obese and diabetic
    D. Anyone with arthralgia and myalgia

12. Patients taking which of these heterocyclic antidepressants may develop weight gain as a side effect of treatment?

    A. Selegiline and amphetamines
    B. Mirazapine or trazodone
    C. Lithium and Prozac
    D. Atomoxetine and sertraline

13. The health care practitioner explains to the patient scheduled for an endoscopy that which of these medications will be used to relieve anxiety and provide sedation, light anesthesia, and amnesia during the procedure?

    A. Amphetamine (Adderall)
    B. Glycopyrrolate (Robinul)
    C. Midazolam (Versed)
    D. Buspirone (BuSpar)

14. Antipsychotic medications are useful for treatment of

    A. dementia-related psychosis
    B. nausea and vomiting
    C. attention-deficit disorder with hyperactivity
    D. tardive dyskinesia

15. What class of antipsychotics differs from typical antipsychotics by blocking both serotonin and dopamine receptors and has less potential adverse effects?

    A. Anxiolytics.
    B. Antiemetics.
    C. Antiparkinson's drugs.
    D. Atypical antipsychotics.

16. Treatment of chronic alcoholism in an intensive in-house rehabilitation program includes:

    A. Administration of thiamine, multiple vitamins, and folic acid.
    B. Individual psychotherapy
    C. Administration of caffeine
    D. Promotion of low-protein, high-carbohydrate diet

17. One treatment for alcoholism and/or opiate abuse includes the daily use of maintenance doses of naltrexone which is ordered. The health care practitioner understands that this treatment is ordered:

    A. While the patient is still drinking alcohol to aid in the elimination of excess dopamine released by drinking alcohol.
    B. Right after the patient is admitted to the detoxification facility to improve alertness.
    C. To keep alcoholics sober after detoxification by robbing the alcohol or drugs ingested of the pleasurable effects.
    D. To prevent a secondary bacterial infection due to decreased immune response in a debilitated patient.

18. The street names "Crystal," "Crank," "Meth," "Speed" are examples of:

    A. Benzodiazepines.
    B. Methamphetamines.
    C. Marijuana.
    D. Hallucinogens.

19. Which of these actions is correct for the health care practitioner to take if substance abuse is suspected in the workplace?

    A. Report to the person in authority.
    B. Report to the police department.
    C. Talk to the individual to encourage him or her to stop.
    D. Ask colleagues to form an intervention group to talk to the individual.

Matching A

Match the medication listed in Column A with the category listed in Column B. Note that the choices in Column B can be used more than once.

COLUMN A	COLUMN B
_____ 1. Prozac, Zoloft, Celexa	A. CNS stimulants
_____ 2. Vistaril, BuSpar	B. Tricyclic antidepressants
_____ 3. Xanax, Ativan, Serax	C. MAO inhibitors
_____ 4. Lithium, Tegretol, Depakene	D. Selective MAO inhibitor
_____ 5. Selegilene	E. Anxiolytics (benzodiazepines)
_____ 6. Thorazine, Haldol, Compazine	F. Anxiolytics (non-benzodiazepines)
_____ 7. Cafcit, Ritalin, Adderall	G. Antipsychotic (typical)
_____ 8. Versed	H. Antipsychotic (atypical)
_____ 9. Lexapro, Paxil, Effexor	I. SSRIs
_____ 10. Elavil, Toframil, Sinequan	J. non-stimulant
_____ 11. Seroquel, Risperdal, Geodon	K. Heterocyclic antidepressants
_____ 12. Nardil, Marplan	L. Antimanic agents
_____ 13. Valium	
_____ 14. Zyprexa, Clozaril, Abilify	
_____ 15. Wellbutrin, Remeron, Desyrel	
_____ 16. Strattera	

Matching B

Match the description in Column A with the terms listed in Column B.

COLUMN A	COLUMN B
_____ 1. Classified as a CNS depressant, also provides properties of a euphoriant, sedative, and hallucinogen	A. Addiction
_____ 2. An inability to coordinate muscle activity during voluntary movement	B. Chemical dependency

(Matching continued on next page)

COLUMN A (continued)	COLUMN B (continued)

_____ 3. Alcohol and/or drugs have taken control of an individual's life and affect normal functioning

C. Habituation

_____ 4. Produce bizarre mental reactions and distortion of physical senses; hallucinations and delusions are common

D. Amphetamines

_____ 5. Psychological dependence only

E. Ataxia

_____ 6. Can be produced and prescribed legally or produced illegally; provides pleasant mental stimulation

F. Cocaine

_____ 7. Consists of tolerance, psychological dependence, physical dependence, and withdrawal reaction with physiological effects

G. Hallucinogens

_____ 8. A CNS stimulant and produces euphoria and increased expenditure of energy; only legal form is topical local anesthetic

H. Marijuana

True or False

Circle T for true or F for false after reading each of the following statements.

1. T F   Use of CNS stimulants in the treatment of obesity is not recommended.

2. T F   CNS stimulants are contraindicated in patients with a history of drug dependence, alcoholism, or eating disorders.

3. T F   The tricyclics have an immediate action; the patient typically reports improved mood and increasing alertness within 2–4 days.

4. T F   Side effects of MAO inhibitors are adrenergic in action and can include nervousness, agitation, insomnia, and hypertension or hypertensive crisis.

5. T F   Treatment of depression with SSRIs is preferred because of increased compliance and fewer side effects.

6. T F   Regular monitoring of temperature is important in patients receiving the SSRI Effexor.

7. T F   There is a possibility of drug interaction when SSRIs are taken MAIOs.

8. T F   Atomoxetine (Strattera) is a selective norepinephrine reuptake inhibitor (SNRI) noncontrolled drug used for attention-deficit hyperactivity disorder.

9. T F   Symbyax, a combination of the atypical antipsychotic olanzapine and the SSRI fluoxetine, is the first FDA-approved combination product for the depressive phase of bipolar disorder.

10. T F   Polyuria and thirst are side effects of the antimanic drug lithium and can lead to dehydration, causing acute toxicity.

11. T F   If trazodone, a heterocyclic antidepressant, causes a priapism or impotence, it should be discontinued.

12. T F   Increased respirations and agitation with large doses, occur with the administration of the anxiolytic midazolam (Versed), especially in older adults and those with COPD.

13. T F   Vistaril and Atarax are short-term anxiolytics; however, they are chemically different than the benzodiazepines.

14. T F   Antipsychotic medications are also called neuroleptics.

15. T F   Patients taking atypical antipsychotics are at increased risk for hyperglycemia and diabetes.

16. T F Patients taking the atypical antipsychotics clozapine (Clozaril) and olanzapine (Zyprexa) have a possible side effect of severe weight loss.

17. T F Haloperidol (Haldol) is a typical antipsychotic prescribed for agitation and delusions.

18. T F Alcohol (ethyl alcohol, ethanol) can be classified as a psychotropic drug and a CNS stimulant.

19. T F A reduced risk of myocardial infarction has been noted in research when an individual consumed one to two drinks of wine per day (5–6 days each week) as compared with nondrinkers.

20. T F If naltrexone is given to someone currently dependent on opiates, it can send the addict instantly into severe, life-threatening withdrawal.

21. T F Prescription drugs most often abused by medical personnel are hydrocodone, oxycodone, and the benzodiazepines.

22. T F Acute toxicity from amphetamines can include severe cardiovascular symptoms such as circulatory collapse, along with confusion, delirium, belligerence, and suicidal or homicidal tendencies.

23. T F Treatment of amphetamine overdosage consists of administration of the specific antidote usually prescribed for overdosage.

24. T F Cocaine has been approved for medical use as a local anesthetic normally used topically for nasal procedures.

Case Study

Nancy Wood comes to your office to see the doctor about a recent panic attack. She stated that she felt like the walls of her friend's apartment were closing in on her, her heart was pounding, she was sweating, and she felt like she had no air to breathe.

1. Which of these classes of drugs used for panic disorder is considered the safest because of low occurrence of side effects and lack of physiological dependence?

   A. Tricyclics
   B. Benzodiazepines
   C. Monoamine oxidase inhibitors
   D. Selective serotonin reuptake inhibitors

2. After the physician orders alprazolam (Xanax XR), the health care practitioner should teach the patient to

   A. Avoid taking medication with grapefruit juice.
   B. Take the pulse before swallowing medication.
   C. Have white blood cell counts drawn at the lab every 6 weeks.
   D. Observe for signs of jaundice.

3. The health care practitioner should be alert for any indication that this patient

   A. Does not understands the dietary restrictions
   B. Has difficulty sleeping
   C. Develops urinary retention
   D. Is experiencing hair loss

4. The health care practitioner should instruct the patient to

   A. discontinue the medication immediately if a rash develops.
   B. take an additional dose of medication if symptom are not relieved immediately.
   C. avoid stopping the medication abruptly.
   D. report any signs of drowsiness.

CHAPTER 21

Musculoskeletal and Anti-Inflammatory Drugs

Fill-in-the-Blank

Fill in the blank for each of the following statements.

1. The health care practitioner understands that most muscle relaxant drugs affect the _____ _____ and the brain, resulting in reduction of muscle spasm, altered perception of pain, and a sedative effect.

2. Muscle relaxant drugs are _____ in pregnant or lactating females and those individuals with myasthenia gravis.

3. Muscle relaxant medications should be taken only as long as absolutely necessary because prolonged use can lead to physical and _____ dependence and withdrawal symptoms.

4. Prolonged use of NSAIDs by older adults and debilitated patients can lead to _____ GI events.

5. If a patient who has developed GI complications related to taking anti-inflammatory medications but requires continued therapy, combination products are available which protects the gastric mucosa, such as _____, a combination of diclofenac (Voltaren) and misoprostol (Cytotec).

6. Nonsteroidal anti-inflammatory medications are _____ in patients with thyroid disease or a history of GI ulcer or inflammatory bowel disease.

7. Celecoxib (Celebrex) is a nonsteroidal anti-inflammatory that acts by _____ inhibiting COX-2 prostaglandin synthesis.

8. Children with viral infections should not be given salicylates due to the danger of developing _____ syndrome.

9. Nonsteroidal anti-inflammatory medications should be administered with _____ or _____ to reduce the GI side effects.

10. Nonsteroidal anti-inflammatory agents, especially salicylates, interact with alcohol and anticoagulants to potentiate the possibility of GI _____.

11. Health care practitioners must be aware that _____ administered with NSAIDs may potentiate hypoglycemia in the patient taking one of these oral hypoglycemic agents.

12. The health care practitioner teaches the patient with gouty arthritis to drink large amounts of fluids when taking _____.

13. Nonsteroidal anti-inflammatory medications (NSAIDs) that inhibit the synthesis of _____ are called nonselective (traditional) NSAIDS.

14. Patients taking NSAIDs should be instructed to avoid taking _____ because of the increase in adverse GI effects.

15. Patients taking bisphosphonates should be instructed by the health care practitioner to take supplemental _____ and _____ _____ and to participate in weight-bearing exercises.

Multiple Choice

Circle the letter that best answers the question.

1. Acute painful musculoskeletal conditions of the back or neck are initially treated with:

   A. Hot or cold packs and mild analgesics.
   B. Corticosteroid injections.
   C. Muscle relaxants, rest, hot and cold packs, and mild analgesics.
   D. Selective COX-2 inhibitor for short-term use followed by corticosteroids for the next 6 months.

2. A muscle relaxant used for spasticity resulting from upper neuron disorders such as occurs with multiple sclerosis or cerebral palsy is called:

   A. Dantrolene (Dantrium).
   B. Carisoprodol (Soma).
   C. Methocarbamol (Robaxin).
   D. Diazepam (Valium).

3. Which of these neuromuscular blocking agents provides muscle relaxation during surgical, endoscopic, or orthopedic procedures and is administered only by anesthesiologists or specially trained personnel skilled in intubation and cardiopulmonary resuscitation?

   A. Cyclobenzaprine (Flexeril)
   B. Diazepam (Valium)
   C. Succinylcholine
   D. Dantrolene

4. Which of these medications is an antidote for the neuromuscular blocking agents?

   A. Neostigmine (Prostigmin)
   B. Rocuronium (Zemeron)
   C. Diclofenac (Voltaren)
   D. Dantrolene (Dantrium)

5. Muscle relaxants must be used with caution in patients with a history of:

   A. Sexual dysfunction.
   B. Back or neck pain.
   C. Gastroesophageal reflux disease.
   D. Drug abuse or liver disorders.

6. Which anti-inflammatory drugs are used to treat arthritis, bursitis, spondylitis, gout, and muscle strains and sprains?

   A. Naproxen (Naprosyn) and indomethacin (Indocin)
   B. Corticosteroids
   C. Diazepam (Valium) and cyclobenzaprine (Flexeril)
   D. Tizandine (Zanaflex) and diclofenac (Voltaren)

7. What substances are responsible for the production of inflammation and pain of rheumatic conditions, sprains, and menstrual cramps?

   A. Salicylates
   B. Endorphin inhibitors
   C. Prostaglandins
   D. Histamines

8. Patients needing prolonged anti-inflammatory therapy after experiencing GI ulceration and bleeding can be switched to a partially *selective NSAID* such as:

   A. Prevacid.
   B. Arthrotec.
   C. Celebrex.
   D. Meloxicam.

9. Patients who have experienced GI ulceration and bleeding but still required prolonged anti-inflammatory therapy can also be switched to a COX-2 inhibitor such as:

   A. Meloxicam.
   B. Etodolac (Lodine).
   C. Arthrotec.
   D. Celebrex.

10. Both traditional NSAIDS and the COX-2s can increase the risk of adverse events in patients who are at risk for which of these conditions?

    A. Bronchitis
    B. Cardiovascular disease
    C. GERD
    D. Parkinson's disease

11. The health care practitioner will assess patients taking which of these medications for prolonged bleeding time, blood dyscrasias, and epigastric pain?

    A. COX-2 inhibitors
    B. Muscle relaxants
    C. Benzodiazepines
    D. NSAIDs

12. The health care practitioner explains to the patient who has just been diagnosed with gout that it is a metabolic disorder manifested by swelling and pain due to accumulation of uric acid crystals in joints, especially the:

    A. Shoulder and neck.
    B. Hip and shoulder.
    C. Big toe, ankle, knee, and elbow.
    D. Hip, knee, shoulder, and wrist.

13. The health care practitioner teaches patients taking NSAIDs to discontinue the drug and report to physician if which of these occurs?

    A. Pruritus
    B. Epigastric pain or nausea
    C. Constipation
    D. Knee or hip pain

14. Patients taking bisphosphonates such Fosamax or Actonel should be instructed to take medication with a full glass of water:

    A. In the morning at least 30 minutes prior to eating food, drinking a beverage, or taking another medication.
    B. At least 1 hour after the midday meal, then lie down for approximately 30 minutes.
    C. At bedtime with food to avoid irritation of the stomach.
    D. In the evening just after eating.

Matching A

Match the generic name of the muscle relaxant listed in Column A with the trade name listed in Column B

COLUMN A	COLUMN B
_____ 1. Baclofen	A. Valium
_____ 2. Carisoprodol	B. Soma
_____ 3. Cyclobenzaprine	C. Robaxin
_____ 4. Dantrolene	D. Lioresal
_____ 5. Diazepam	E. Dantrium
_____ 6. Methocarbamol	F. Flexeril
_____ 7. Tizanidine	G. Zanaflex

Matching B

Match the anti-inflammatory medication listed in Column A with the category listed in Column B. Note that the choices in Column B can be used more than once.

COLUMN A	COLUMN B
_____ 1. Diclofenac (Voltaren)	A. Gout medications
_____ 2. Diclofenac/misoprostol	B. Combinations (NSAID / GI protectant)
_____ 3. Colchicine	C. Selective COX-2 inhibitors
_____ 4. Ketorolac (Toradol)	D. Partially selective NSAIDs
_____ 5. Etodolac (Lodine)	E. Nonselective NSAIDS
_____ 6. Indomethacin (Indocin)	
_____ 7. Naproxen (Aleve, Anaprox)	
_____ 8. Celecoxib (Celebrex)	
_____ 9. Meloxicam (Mobic)	
_____ 10. Lansoprazole/naproxen (Prevacid NapraPAC)	
_____ 11. Nabumetone (Relafen)	

True or False

Circle T for true or F for false after reading each of the following statements.

1. T F Muscle relaxants are contraindicated in patients with muscular dystrophy and children under 12 years of age.

2. T F Analgesics and psychotrophic medications interact with muscle relaxants to decrease their effect.

3. T F Patients needing prolonged anti-inflammatory therapy after experiencing GI ulceration and bleeding can be switched to a partially selective NSAID, a selective COX-2 inhibitor, or a combination product (NSAID plus drug that inhibits gastric acid).

4. T F NSAIDs should be discontinued 10–14 days before elective surgery or dental procedures to reduce the risk of serious bleeding.

5. T F Patients allergic to sulfa should not take Celebrex.

6. T F Colchicine is also used as a prophylaxis in persons prone to gouty arthritis.

7. T   F   The health care practitioner is responsible for staying informed of the latest developments related to the NSAIDs, specifically the COX-2 inhibitors, by checking on the FDA Web site.

8. T   F   Raloxifene (Evista) is the drug of choice during pregnancy and in women with a history of thromboembolic disorders as prevention of osteoporosis.

9. T   F   Calcitonin is reserved for women who cannot tolerate hormone replacement therapy or in whom it is contraindicated.

10. T   F   Patients taking Fosamax or Actonel should be instructed to avoid lying down at least 30 minutes after taking medications to avoid esophageal irritation.

Case Study

Macy Watts, 75 years old, comes to see the doctor about a possible fracture in her wrist. The physician diagnoses osteoporosis and discusses the possible treatment plans with her.

1. As the health care practitioner, you are aware that osteoporosis is a disease characterized by:

    A. Low bone mass and deterioration of bone tissue.
    B. Collection of uric acid crystals in the joints of the foot.
    C. Muscle spasms of the upper and lower back and neck.
    D. Bone spurs and multiple herniated vertebral disks.

2. The health care practitioner knows that osteoporosis is seen most frequently in which of these groups?

    A. Older men who are unable to exercise daily because of musculoskeletal disorders.
    B. Women who have been taking birth control pills for a prolonged period of time.
    C. Older women, primarily postmenopausal.
    D. Younger men or women with chronic musculoskeletal problems.

3. Hormone replacement therapy (HRT), estrogen with or without progestin, is recommended for prevention of postmenopausal osteoporosis:

    A. Beginning at age 40.
    B. Only when the patient is unable to take other agents.
    C. For patients who have a history of dysmenorrhea.
    D. For patients who are unable to exercise.

4. The health care practitioner explains to this patient that estrogen:

    A. Provides the patient with enough energy to exercise.
    B. Treats postmenopausal osteoporosis for patients 5 years past menopause.
    C. Reverses the aging process that accelerates during the perimenopausal period.
    D. Prevents the accelerated phase of bone loss, which occurs the first 5 years postmenopause.

5. The health care practitioner explains to the patient that therapy with selective estrogen-receptor modifiers, such as Evista, increase bone mineral density and reduce fracture risk without:

    A. Deferring the process of menopause.
    B. Promoting breast or endometrial cancer.
    C. Increasing the potential for weight gain.
    D. Postponing the progression of menopause.

6. The health care practitioner explains to the patient that Miacalcin, a synthetic form of the hormone calcitonin, is administered which of these forms?

    A. Subcutaneous injection
    B. Oral medication
    C. Nasal spray
    D. Rectal suppository

7. Bisphosphonates act directly to inhibit bone resorption, increasing bone mineral density at the spine and hip and decreasing the incidence of first and future fractures and include which of these medications?

   A. Alendronate (Fosamax) and risedronate (Actonel)
   B. Colchicine and indomethacin (Indocin)
   C. Nabumetone (Relafen)
   D. Raloxifene (Evista)

CHAPTER 22

Anticonvulsants, Antiparkinsonian Drugs, and Agents for Alzheimer's Disease

Fill-in-the-Blank

Fill in the blank for each of the following statements.

1. Treatment of epilepsy is based on type, severity, and cause of _____.

2. Grand mal and absence seizures are called _____ seizures because they are bilaterally symmetrical and without local onset.

3. Grand mal (tonic-clonic) seizures typically last two to _____ minutes and are manifested by abrupt loss of consciousness, falling, and possibly urinary and fecal incontinence.

4. When seizures occur so frequently that the patient does not regain consciousness between the seizures, the condition is called _____ _____.

5. The treatment of choice for the patient experiencing status epilepticus is lorazepam (_____) administered intravenously.

6. Initial treatment for a patient experiencing a grand mal seizure consists only of _____ _____ by removing any objects that could cause trauma, turn the head to the side, and loosen tight clothing.

7. Absence epilepsy was previously called _____ _____ epilepsy.

8. Valproic acid (Depakene) is considered a _____ - _____ anticonvulsant.

9. The goal of anticonvulsant therapy is to prevent seizures without _____.

10. The dosage of anticonvulsants is regulated or adjusted according to the individual patient's _____.

11. Possible side effects of phenytoin include headache, sedation, _____, and dizziness.

12. Anticonvulsant therapy may have adverse effects on behavior and _____ in children, especially phenobarbital, phenytoin, and carbamazepine.

13. Sinemet, a combination of levodopa and _____, is most often used for long-term treatment of Parkinson's disease.

14. Sinemet is recommended as initial drug therapy for those over _____ years of age and those with dementia.

15. Patients receiving Sinemet for prolonged periods of time may develop a tolerance, resulting in drug ineffectiveness called "_____ - _____".

16. Side effects of Symmetrel are usually dose related and _____.

17. Aricept, Exelon, Cognex, and Reminyl are agents used in the treatment of Alzheimer's disease and all are _____ inhibitors.

18. Drugs used to treat primary restless legs syndrome (RLS) include dopamine agonists, benzodiazepines, and _____ such as hydrocodone.

Multiple Choice

Circle the letter that best answers the question.

1. Treatment for absence epilepsy includes which of these anticonvulsants?

   A. Gabapentin (Neurontin) and topiramate (Topamax)
   B. Valium and clonazepam (Klonopin)
   C. Valproic acid (Depakene), clonazepam (Klonopin), and ethosuximide (Zarontin)
   D. Corticosteroid injections, Valium, phenytoin (Dilantin), and carbamazepine (Tegretol)

2. Absence seizures typically occur in which of these groups?

   A. Older adults
   B. Only females
   C. Only males
   D. Children

3. Less than half of epileptic seizures have an identifiable cause, such as

   A. coronary heart disease.
   B. hepatitis.
   C. Parkinson's disease.
   D. cerebral trauma.

4. Which of these symptoms are observed in patients who have temporal lobe seizures?

   A. Convulsions
   B. Confusion and impaired judgment
   C. Unilateral tonic-clonic contractions
   D. Urinary incontinence

5. Which of these medications are used for prophylactic treatment of generalized and partial seizures?

   A. Phenytoin (Dilantin), frequently combined with phenobarbital or valproic acid
   B. Clonazepam (Klonopin) combined with valium or ethosuximide (Zarontin)
   C. Gabapentin (Neurontin) and topiramate (Topamax)
   D. Valium and clonazepam (Klonopin)

6. Stevens-Johnson syndrome is a side effect of which anticonvulsant?

   A. Clonazepam (Klonopin)
   B. Topiramate (Topamax)
   C. Phenytoin (Dilantin)
   D. Valproic acid (Depakene)

7. For febrile seizures in children, what is the current treatment recommended by the American Academy of Pediatrics?

    A. Rectal diazepam gel for seizures lasting more than 5 minutes
    B. Oral phenobarbital alone
    C. Oral phenytoin alone
    D. Intravenous fosphenytoin

8. What is a major advantage of second-generation anticonvulsants?

    A. Increased efficacy of seizure control
    B. Drug level monitoring of therapeutic levels is usually not required
    C. Dosages can be decreased
    D. Increased availability of these medications

9. Second-generation anticonvulsants indicated for adjuvant treatment of partial and generalized seizures include:

    A. Tegretol and Neurontin.
    B. Neurontin and Lamictal.
    C. Lamictal and Klonopin.
    D. Klonopin and Tegretol.

10. Which of these instructions should be given to patients taking anticonvulsant medications?

    A. Wear a Medic-Alert tag or bracelet at all times in case of accident or injury
    B. Take medication with grapefruit juice
    C. Omit medication if experiencing nausea or upset stomach
    D. Use a hard bristle toothbrush to keep teeth and gums clean

11. When Sinemet is prescribed for patients who have Parkinson's disease, the health care practitioner should observe them for which of these side effects?

    A. GI ulceration and bleeding
    B. Nausea, vomiting, and anorexia
    C. Dyskinesias, behavior changes, and psychosis
    D. Hypertension and depression in male patients

12. Parkinson-like tremors associated with long-term use of antipsychotics are treated with synthetic atropine-like drugs such as:

    A. Levodopa and carbidopa (Sinemet).
    B. Entacapone (Comtan).
    C. Benztropine (Cogentin).
    D. Pramipexole (Mirapex).

13. Which of these antiparkinsonian drugs are dopamine agonists used in conjunction with levodopa to delay the onset of levodopa-caused motor complications?

    A. Anticholinergic agents
    B. Bromocriptine (Parlodel)
    C. Sinemet CR
    D. Benztropine (Cogentin)

14. The health care practitioner explains to patients taking cholinesterase inhibitors such as donepezil (Aricept) that which of these side effects may occur?

    A. Hepatotoxicity
    B. GI upset, nausea, vomiting, and anorexia
    C. Pain in the knee and elbow
    D. Orthostatic hypotension

15. Which of these medications is the first N-methyl-D-aspartate (NMDA) antagonist approved for the treatment of moderate-to-severe dementia of the Alzheimer's type?

   A. Memantine (Namenda)
   B. Donepezil (Aricept)
   C. Tacrine (Cognex)
   D. Galantamine (Reminyl)

16. Restless legs syndrome (RSL) can be primary, involving the central nervous system, or secondary, related to other causes such as

   A. iron deficiency
   B. Parkinson's disease
   C. hyperthyroidism
   D. vitamin C deficiency

Matching A

Match the key term listed in Column A with the description listed in Column B.

COLUMN A	COLUMN B
____ 1. Absence epilepsy	A. Bilateral symmetrical seizures without local onset
____ 2. Anticholinergics	B. Previously called petit mal, 10–30 second loss of consciousness with no falling
____ 3. Anticonvulsants	
____ 4. Epilepsy	C. Tonic, clonic and tonic-clonic seizures with loss of consciousness and control of bodily functions
____ 5. Convulsive seizures	D. Temporal lobe or psychomotor seizures with complex symptomatology
____ 6. Mixed seizure	
____ 7. Alzheimer's disease	E. Used to reduce the number and/or severity of seizures in patients with epilepsy
____ 8. Unilateral seizures	F. Progressive decline in cognitive function with increasingly severe impairment in social and occupational functioning
____ 9. Temporal lobe seizures	
____ 10. Parkinson's disease	G. Recurrence of unprovoked seizures
____ 11. Partial seizures	H. Seizures caused by a lesion in the temporal lobe of the brain
____ 12. Generalized seizures	I. Atropine-like drugs administered to patients with mild forms of drug-induced parkinsonism
	J. Seizures that affect only one side of the body
	K. Combining more than one kind of seizure pattern
	L. Chronic neurologic disorder characterized by fine, slowly spreading muscle tremors, rigidity, and weakness of muscles and shuffling gait

Matching B

Match the anticonvulsant trade name listed in Column A with the generic name listed in Column B.

COLUMN A	COLUMN B
____ 1. Topamax	A. Carbamazepine
____ 2. Zarontin	B. Valproic acid
____ 3. Neurontin	C. Topiramate
____ 4. Lamictal	D. Gabapentin

_____ 5. Dilantin   E. Clonazepam

_____ 6. Cerebyx   F. Fosphenytoin

_____ 7. Klonopin   G. Phenytoin

_____ 8. Depakene   H. Ethosuximide

_____ 9. Tegretol   I. Lamotrigine

True or False

Circle T for true or F for false after reading each of the following statements.

1. T   F   A patient having an absence seizure will lose consciousness for 10–30 seconds while sitting upright in a chair.

2. T   F   IV phenytoin and lorazepam are given for treatment of status epilepticus.

3. T   F   Patients taking Dilantin may have side effects such as dizziness, sedation, and ataxia, which frequently decrease with continued treatment.

4. T   F   Patients should be instructed not to abruptly discontinue any anticonvulsant medication without consulting the physician who ordered the medication.

5. T   F   Patients should be instructed to take Tegretol with grapefruit juice.

6. T   F   Mixed seizures occur as a combined pattern of more than one type.

7. T   F   The health care practitioner should teach parents of children receiving anticonvulsants to be aware of and report any changes in cognitive function, mood, and behavior.

8. T   F   Careful oral hygiene should be taught to patients taking anticonvulsants until tenderness of the gums subsides as their treatment progresses.

9. T   F   Second-generation anticonvulsants have more side effects and require lab monitoring of therapeutic levels.

10. T   F   Patients taking entacapone should not receive nonselective MAOIs but can take a selective MAOI such as selegiline.

11. T   F   Patients taking a cholinesterase inhibitor for symptom delay in Alzheimer's disease should expect to see improved cognitive function but understand that the disease will not be cured.

12. T   F   The first cholinesterase inhibitor approved was tacrine (Cognex) but is associated with significant hepatotoxicity and a frequent dosing schedule.

Case Study

Gwen Winter, 55 years old, has been diagnosed with Parkinson's disease. She has concerns and questions about her medication regime.

1. The health care practitioner knows that Parkinson's disease is characterized by:

   A. Continuous seizures without regaining consciousness between the seizures.
   B. Fine, slowly spreading muscle tremors, rigidity, and weakness of muscles and shuffling gait.
   C. Progressive decline in cognitive function with increasingly severe impairment in social and occupational functioning.
   D. Recurrent paroxymal disorder of brain function characterized by sudden attacks of altered consciousness, motor activity, or sensory impairment.

2. The health care practitioner explains to the patient that Parkinson's disease:

   A. Is a temporary disorder affecting her ability to exercise daily.
   B. Does not have a cure, but that she will not get any worse over time.
   C. Has no cure and, as the disease advances, she may develop declining cognitive function.
   D. Has neuromuscular alterations that will be corrected by the correct medication.

3. What is the treatment goal for patients who have Parkinson's disease?

   A. Relieve symptoms and maintain mobility.
   B. Control seizures without oversedation.
   C. Relieve the cholinergic systems and improve function.
   D. Provide the patient with enough energy to exercise.

4. The health care practitioner explains to the patient that levodopa crosses the blood-brain barrier where it is converted to:

   A. Acetylcholine.
   B. Serotonin.
   C. Dopamine.
   D. Epinephrine.

5. The health care practitioner explains to the patient that combining levodopa and carbidopa in one medication:

   A. Defers the process of neurotransmitters at the synapse.
   B. Promotes the cholinergic effect.
   C. Increases the therapeutic effect of dopamine in the CNS and reduces its adverse reactions.
   D. Postpones in the progression of the nerve impulses and therefore reduces the adverse reactions.

6. The health care practitioner explains to the patient that catechol-O-methyltransferase (COMT) inhibitors allows the patient's dose of levodopa to be lowered and decreases the incidence and/or severity of levodopa dose-related side effects. Which of these medications is a COMT inhibitor?

   A. Ropinirole (Requip)
   B. Entacapone (Comtan)
   C. Benztropine (Cogentin)
   D. Trihexyphenidyl (Artane)

7. Which information should the health care practitioner teach the patient about antiparkinsonian drugs?

   A. Take the prescribed medications on as "as needed" basis.
   B. Stop the medication if side effects occur.
   C. Tell the physician if the medication is not effective after 24 hours.
   D. Maintain physical activity, self-care, and social interaction.

CHAPTER 23

Endocrine System Drugs

Fill-in-the-Blank

Fill in the blank for each of the following statements.

1. The endocrine system drugs include natural _____ secreted by the ductless glands or synthetic substitutes.

2. The pituitary gland is located at the base of the _____.

3. The _____ gland is called the master gland because it regulates the function of the other glands.

4. The anterior pituitary lobe hormone, _____, is called human growth hormone (HGH).

5. Adrenocorticotropic hormone (ACTH) is available only for _____ use as corticotrophin and is used mainly for adrenocortical insufficiency.

6. The use of _____ can be subdivided into two categories: one as replacement therapy when the patient has a deficit in secretions, and the other for their anti-inflammatory and immunosuppressant properties.

7. Corticosteroids are used with other _____ drugs to prevent rejection of transplanted organs.

8. Health care practitioners must teach patients beginning on a corticosteroid that prolonged use will result in _____ of the pituitary gland, ending the body's normal secretion of corticosteroids.

9. The health care practitioner should caution patients that corticosteroids must be withdrawn _____ and not abruptly stopped, to allow the pituitary gland to resume its normal functioning.

10. For patients on corticosteroid therapy, administering vaccines and toxoids will _____ the antibody response.

11. Patients taking corticosteroids beyond very brief periods may have delayed wound healing and increased _____ to infection.

12. An adverse effect of corticosteroid therapy in older women is development of _____ with fractures.

13. Hypothyroidism is diagnosed by blood tests such as TSH _____ medication is given.

14. Patients suffering from hypothyroidism have _____ metabolism with symptoms ranging from fatigue, dry skin, weight gain, sensitivity to cold, and irregular menses to mental retardation if untreated.

15. Thyroid replacement therapy for true hypothyroidism must be continued for _____, although dosage adjustments may be required.

16. It is essential that the health care practitioner administering levothyroxine check the dosage ordered and note the decimal place (0.025 mg vs 0.25 mg) when converting between mg and mcg to avoid a _____ _____.

17. Health care practitioners must be able to describe the differences in insulin preparations according to their onset, _____, and duration of action.

18. When the physician orders insulin individualized on a _____ _____ scale, the amount administered is based on the blood glucose level assessed just before giving the insulin, typically ordered before meals and at bedtime.

19. When two insulins are ordered at the same time, _____ insulin should always be drawn into the syringe first, then the intermediate or long acting insulin.

20. Unopened insulin vials should not be subjected to _____.

Multiple Choice

Circle the letter that best answers the question.

1. The hormones that act on the immune system to suppress the body's response to infection or trauma and relieve inflammation are called:

    A. Thyroid hormones.
    B. Neurotransmitters.
    C. Corticosteroids.
    D. Adrenergics.

2. When patients are on corticosteroids for extended duration, serious side effects may occur, such as:

    A. Decreased intraocular pressure.
    B. Osteoporosis with fractures, especially in older women.
    C. Heart attack.
    D. Decreased serum sodium.

3. Corticosteroids are contraindicated in which of the following patients?

    A. A 21-year-old with poison ivy
    B. A 37-year-old with status asthmaticus
    C. A 50-year-old car wreck victim with cerebral edema
    D. A 30-year-old with nonlife-threatening bacterial infection

4. When corticosteroids are administered to a patient who has diabetes, the health care practitioner would expect the blood glucose level to:

    A. Slowly decrease.
    B. Rapidly decrease to a state of hypoglycemia.
    C. Increase to a state of hyperglycemia.
    D. Remain normal unless the patient has an infection.

5. Which of these medications increase the effects of corticosteroids?

    A. Estrogens and oral contraceptives
    B. Antacids and phenytoin (Dilantin)
    C. Rifampin and carbamazepine
    D. Cholestyramine and meperidine

6. Which of these toxic side effects would the health care practitioner observe in a patient who is taking a thyroid agent for treatment of hypothyroidism?

    A. Hypertension, tachycardia, and nervousness
    B. Hypotension, bradycardia, and hypoglycemia
    C. Muscle cramps, weakness, and constriction of the pupils
    D. Jaundice, hypotension, and sweating

7. Which of these antithyroid agents are used to relieve the symptoms of hyperthyroidism in preparation for surgical or radioactive iodine therapy?

   A. Levothyroxine and methylprednisolone
   B. Dexamethasone and corticotrophin
   C. Tapazole and propylthiouracil
   D. Corticotropin and levothyroxine

8. Prior to administering insulin, the health care practitioner should always have someone else check:

   A. The dosage ordered with the insulin drawn up in the syringe in order to prevent a medication error.
   B. The syringe to verify that it is a U-100 syringe marked so that each unit represents 2 units.
   C. To see if the patient has eaten since the last dosage of insulin.
   D. For any signs of hypoglycemia or hyperglycemia in the patient.

9. Which insulin preparation should not be mixed with any of the other available types of insulin?

   A. Regular insulin
   B. Lispro (Humalog)
   C. Lente (Humulin L)
   D. Glargine (Lantus)

10. Which one of these insulins has an onset of action within 15 minutes?

    A. Glargine (Lantus)
    B. Humulin R
    C. Humalog
    D. Humulin N

11. Which one of the following insulins has no pronounced peak of action?

    A. Regular (Humulin R)
    B. Glargine (Lantus)
    C. Aspart (NovoLog)
    D. Isophane (Novolin N)

12. When teaching the patient and family about insulin, the health care practitioner will advise that open vials of insulin may be stored at room temperature without loss of potency for:

    A. One hour.
    B. One day.
    C. 14 days.
    D. 28 days.

13. Which of these insulins have peak action of 30 minutes to 1 hour and last for approximately 3 hours?

    A. Humulin R and Novolin R
    B. Humalog and NovoLog
    C. Novolin N and Humulin N
    D. Levemir and Lantus

14. The health care practitioner should teach the patient with diabetes and the patient's family that hyperglycemia may result from:

    A. Infections or emotional stress.
    B. Overdose of insulin.
    C. Delayed or insufficient food intake.
    D. Excessive or unusual exercise.

15. Symptoms of hyperglycemia include:

    A. Increased perspiration and/or tingling of the fingers
    B. Irritability, confusion, or bizarre behavior
    C. Dehydration and excessive thirst
    D. Tremor, headache, and weakness

16. The health care practitioner should teach the patient and family that hypoglycemia may result from:

    A. Infections or emotional stress.
    B. Surgical or other trauma.
    C. Overdose of insulin and insufficient food intake.
    D. Insufficient dose of insulin and excessive carbohydrate intake.

17. Symptoms of hypoglycemia include:

    A. Irritability, confusion, or bizarre behavior
    B. Vision problems and excessive urination
    C. Dehydration and excessive thirst
    D. Polyuria and anorexia

18. Which of these medications antagonize the action of insulin, necessitating increased insulin dosage?

    A. Alcohol
    B. Salicylates
    C. MAO inhibitors
    D. Corticosteroids

19. Which of these medications interact with insulin to potentiate hypoglycemic effects?

    A. Oral contraceptives and estrogen
    B. Corticosteroids and epinephrine
    C. Salicylates and alcohol
    D. Estrogen and corticosteroids

20. Appropriate treatment of a conscious patient with hypoglycemia includes:

    A. 8 oz of orange juice with five packs of granulated sugar for a conscious patient.
    B. IV fluids to correct electrolyte balance with regular insulin added.
    C. 10–30 mL of 50% dextrose solution IV or administration.
    D. Giving a large dose of insulin and then getting a physician's order to administer a corticosteroid followed by a protein snack.

21. If the physician orders metformin (Glucophage) for a patient who has Type 2 diabetes, the patient should be taught that this medication falls into which category of oral antidiabetic agents?

    A. Biguanides
    B. Alpha-glucosidase inhibitors
    C. Meglitinides
    D. Thiazolidinediones

22. Metformin (Glucophage) works by:

    A. Delaying digestion of carbohydrates and subsequent absorption of glucose.
    B. Decreasing hepatic glucose output and enhancing insulin sensitivity in muscle.
    C. Decreasing insulin resistance/improving sensitivity to insulin in muscle and adipose tissue.
    D. Stimulating insulin production from the pancreas and improving peripheral insulin activity.

23. If a patient who is taking metformin (Glucophage) is scheduled for a special diagnostic procedure requiring contrast media, the health care practitioner should instruct the patient to hold this medication the day of the procedure and for how long following completion of the procedure?

    A. No further delay is necessary
    B. 24 hours
    C. 48 hours
    D. One week

24. Repaglinide (Prandin), which stimulates beta cells of the pancreas to produce insulin and can be used as monotherapy or in combination with metformin, is categorized as a

    A. Thiazolidinedione.
    B. Meglitinide.
    C. Sulfonylurea.
    D. Biguanide.

25. The patient taking repaglinide (Prandin) should be instructed to take the medication:

    A. After meals to decrease the GI effects.
    B. At bedtime at least 2 hours after eating.
    C. At least 1 hour before breakfast.
    D. Before meals to maximize the absorption.

26. Which of these medications can be ordered to lower blood glucose in a patient who has insulin resistant Type 2 diabetes by decreasing insulin resistance and improving sensitivity to insulin in muscle and adipose tissue?

    A. Prandin or Starlix
    B. Actos or Avandia
    C. Metformin or Precose
    D. Glipizide or Glyburide

27. When teaching patients who are learning to self-administer insulin, it is important for patients to understand which information about injection sites is true?

    A. All sites have the same absorption rate whether exercising or not.
    B. Insulin injected into the abdomen will be absorbed least consistently.
    C. Insulin injected into the arm or thigh is absorbed less rapidly than in the abdomen.
    D. Exercise will increase absorption, especially when insulin is injected in the arm or thigh.

28. Which insulin is to be drawn into the syringe first if regular insulin is to be mixed with NPH?

    A. It does not make any difference.
    B. NPH cannot be mixed with any other insulin.
    C. Draw up the regular first.
    D. Draw up the NPH first.

29. Which of these factors could affect the blood glucose level sufficiently to decrease the amount of insulin a patient is required to takes?

    A. Increased stress
    B. Trauma or illness
    C. Increased regular exercise
    D. Increased amount of food intake

Matching A

Match the hormone listed in Column A with the gland that secretes the hormone listed in Column B. Note that the choices in Column B can be used more than once.

COLUMN A	COLUMN B
_____ 1. Corticosteroids	A. Adrenal
_____ 2. Gonadotropic hormones (FSH, LH, LTH)	B. Islet of Langerhans in the pancreas
_____ 3. Insulin	C. Pituitary
_____ 4. Thyroid-stimulating hormone (TSH)	
_____ 5. Somatotropin	
_____ 6. Adrenocorticotropic hormone (ACTH)	

Matching B

Match the generic name of the medication listed in Column A with the trade name listed in Column B.

COLUMN A	COLUMN B
_____ 1. Methylprednisolone	A. Decadron
_____ 2. Cosyntropin	B. Tapazole
_____ 3. Levothyroxine	C. H.P. Acthar Gel
_____ 4. Propylthiouracil	D. PTU
_____ 5. Triamcinolone	E. Cortrosyn
_____ 6. Dexamethasone	F. Synthroid
_____ 7. Corticotropin (ACTH)	G. Solu-Cortef
_____ 8. Methimazole	H. Solu-Medrol
_____ 9. Thyroid	I. Kenalog
_____ 10. Hydrocortisone	J. Armour Thyroid

Matching C

Match the preparation and trade name listed in Column A with the insulin type/action listed in Column B. Note that the choices in Column B can be used more than once.

COLUMN A	COLUMN B
_____ 1. NPH/Reg, Humulin/Novolin	A. Mixtures
_____ 2. Levemir	B. Intermediate
_____ 3. NovoLog	C. Rapid
_____ 4. Humalog	D. Short
_____ 5. Lantus	E. Long
_____ 6. Novolin N	
_____ 7. Humulin R	
_____ 8. Humulin N	
_____ 9. Novolin R	
_____ 10. NPL/Lispro, Humalog Mix 75/25	

Matching D

Match the trade name of the oral antidiabetic agent listed in Column A with the generic name listed in Column B. Note that one of the choices in Column B can be used more than once.

COLUMN A	COLUMN B
_____ 1. Precose	A. Glyburide
_____ 2. Amaryl	B. Acarbose
_____ 3. Glynase	C. Glyburide/metformin
_____ 4. Glucophage	D. Metformin
_____ 5. Starlix	E. Pioglitazone

(*Matching continued on next page*)

COLUMN A (continued)	COLUMN B (continued)
____ 6. Avandia	F. Repaglinide
____ 7. Glucotrol	G. Glimepiride
____ 8. Avandamet	H. Nateglinide
____ 9. Actos	I. Glipizide
____ 10. Glynase	J. Rosiglitazone
____ 11. Glyset	K. Rosiglitazone/metformin
____ 12. Glucovance	L. Miglitol
____ 13. Prandin	

True or False

Circle T for true or F for false after reading each of the following statements.

1. T F Corticosteroid therapy is used for acute flare-ups of severe skin conditions that do not respond to conservative therapy.

2. T F On occasion corticosteroids are used in the cure of malignancies such as leukemia, lymphoma, and Hodgkin's disease.

3. T F In situations of allergic reactions to insect bites, poison plants, chemicals, or other medications with severe symptoms, corticosteroids are often ordered.

4. T F Corticosteroids are often administered to patients for respiratory disorders in order to decrease the inflammatory process and increase the diameter of the airways.

5. T F Treatment for cerebral edema associated with brain trauma or neurosurgery includes corticosteroids to decrease inflammation.

6. T F Health care practitioners must teach parents to observe their child's growth rate when receiving corticosteroid treatment because these drugs may increase the child's rate of growth.

7. T F A side effect of corticosteroid therapy is gastric or esophageal irritation, ulceration, or hemorrhage.

8. T F Corticosteroids will inhibit the antibody response for patients on corticosteroid therapy if they receive vaccines and toxoids.

9. T F Corticosteroids may increase the intraocular pressure in patients with glaucoma and should be administered with extreme caution.

10. T F Hypothyroid conditions requiring replacement therapy include congenital cretinism and adult myxedema.

11. T F A patient with type 2 diabetes mellitus does not produce any insulin.

12. T F Insulin must be administered parenterally because it is destroyed in the GI tract.

13. T F The health care practitioner using a 50 unit (1/2 mL) syringe recognizes that each line represents 1 unit of insulin, and with a 100 U (1 mL) syringe each line represents 2 units of insulin.

14. T F Regular insulin is the only type of insulin that can be given intravenously.

15. T F Hyperglycemic reactions in the older adult may mimic a cerebrovascular accident.

16. T F Combinations of regular and intermediate-acting insulins are also available in the same bottle such as Humulin 70/30.

17. T F Female patients who have Type 2 diabetes should be taught that Actos, an oral antidiabetic agent, can reduce the effectiveness of oral contraceptives.

18. T F Thiazolidinediones such as Avandia may cause weight gain, fluid retention, and/or edema.

Case Study

Eli Jordon, 55 years old, attends the medical clinic once every month. He has just been diagnosed with type 2 diabetes mellitus.

1. What are the symptoms of type 2 diabetes mellitus?

    A. Polydipsia, polyuria, weakness, and poor circulation
    B. Decreased urinary output, weight loss, and euphoria
    C. Bulging eyes and hair loss
    D. Stunted growth and loss of appetite

2. The health care practitioner is aware that type 2 diabetes mellitus can be treated with several types of oral antidiabetic agents individually or in combination. If the physician orders a sulfonylurea for Eli, he will need to understand that it works by:

    A. Delaying digestion of carbohydrates and subsequent absorption of glucose.
    B. Decreasing hepatic glucose output and enhancing insulin sensitivity in muscle.
    C. Decreasing insulin resistance/improving sensitivity to insulin in muscle and adipose tissue.
    D. Stimulating insulin production from the pancreas and improving peripheral insulin activity.

3. The health care practitioner explains that which of these side effects can occur when the patient takes sulfonylureas?

    A. Tachycardia, nervousness, and anginal pain
    B. GI distress, hypoglycemia, and weight gain
    C. Muscle cramps, weakness, and low blood pressure
    D. Jaundice, weight loss, euphoria, decreased sweating

4. The health care practitioner assesses Eli's current medications because there is a possibility that hypoglycemia can be potentiated when which medications are given with sulfonylureas?

    A. Beta-blockers, MAO inhibitors, and Probenecid
    B. Diuretics, phenothiazines, and corticosteroids
    C. Calcium channel blockers
    D. Isoniazid

5. The health care practitioner knows the treatment for type 2 diabetes mellitus will possibly include an alpha-glucosidase inhibitor (Acarbose) along with the sulfonylurea (Glyburide). Alpha-glucosidase inhibitors act to

    A. Delay digestion of complex carbohydrates and subsequent absorption of glucose, resulting in a smaller rise in blood glucose levels following meals.
    B. Decrease insulin resistance/improve sensitivity to insulin in muscle and adipose tissue.
    C. Decrease hepatic glucose output and enhance insulin sensitivity in muscle cells.
    D. Stimulate insulin production from the pancreas and improve peripheral insulin activity.

6. The health care practitioner explains that side effects of Acarbose that may diminish with time or with a reduction in dose are:

    A. Arthralgia and headache.
    B. Flatulence, abdominal distension/pain, and loose stools.
    C. Blood dyscrasias, including anemia.
    D. Dermatologic effects, including rash and pruritus.

CHAPTER 24

Reproductive System Drugs

Fill-in-the-Blank

Fill in the blank for each of the following statements.

1. The male sex hormones secreted in the interstitial tissue of the male testes and the adrenal cortex in both sexes are called _____.

2. Testosterone and andosterone are the androgens responsible for development of _____ sexual characteristics.

3. Androgens are used to treat patients who have hypogonadism or delayed puberty, as replacement when testosterone is diminished, and as _____ treatment for women with advanced metastatic carcinoma of the breast.

4. Androgen therapy is used with caution in prepubertal males because growth may be stunted by premature _____ of bone ends.

5. Androgen therapy can cause an _____ in LDL cholesterol and a _____ in HDL cholesterol.

6. Health care practitioners are responsible to inform athletes, especially adolescents, regarding the hazards of taking the illegal _____ testosterone products to build muscle power or physique.

7. Phosphodiesterase (PDE) inhibitors are a class of drugs given orally for the treatment of male _____ dysfunction.

8. Side effects of PDE inhibitors include headache, flushing, vision abnormalities, with cardiovascular events occurring in less than _____ percent of patients.

9. PDE inhibitors are _____ in older adult patients and patients with preexisting cardiovascular risk factors.

10. Patients taking high doses of estrogen are at _____ _____ for thromboembolic disorders, hypertension, myocardial infarction, and stroke.

11. The health care practitioner should inform the patient taking rifampin or isoniazid that _____ _____ will be ineffective while taking these antitubercular medications.

12. Oral anticoagulant, anticonvulsant, and oral hypoglycemic actions may be _____ when the patient is on estrogen therapy.

13. Synthetic drugs that exert progesterone-like activities are called _____.

14. Progestins are used in the treatment of amenorrhea and abnormal bleeding caused by _____ _____.

15. Synthetic progestins such as _____, are used to treat anorexia, weight loss, and cachexia associated with AIDS.

16. Depo-Provera, 100–500 mg IM weekly to monthly has been used in the management of _____ (sexual deviancy in males), especially for pedophilia and sexual sadism.

17. Progestins are contraindicated in patients with a history of thromboembolic disorders or those that _____, and especially those who have both risk factors.

18. The emergency contraceptive Plan B, if taken within three days of sexual intercourse, prevents _____ or blocks implantation of a fertilized egg.

Multiple Choice

Circle the letter that best answers the question.

1. The health care practitioner should include which information when teaching diabetic patients who are taking androgens and insulin?

   A. Monitor blood sugars carefully because androgens will decrease blood glucose and insulin requirements.
   B. Androgens will stimulate increased production of insulin by the pancreas.
   C. Insulin injections will not be needed while taking androgens.
   D. Side efforts of insulin dosage may increase while taking androgens.

2. All agents in the androgen class are classified by the DEA as:

   A. Controlled substance (C-II).
   B. Controlled substance (C-III).
   C. Legal only for individuals over the age of 21.
   D. Available for purchase over the counter without a prescription.

3. Which of these statements about estrogen therapy is true?

   A. Estrogen therapy alone is effective for prevention of disease in women who have had a hysterectomy.
   B. The larger the dose of estrogren or combined estrogen/progestin, the more effective relief of menopausal symptoms.
   C. Combined estrogen/progestin therapy should not be used for prevention of cardiovascular disease.
   D. Estrogen therapy is advised for postmenopausal prevention of osteoporosis.

4. The health care practitioner should teach postmenopausal women taking estrogen that one potential side effect is folic acid deficiency to increase their dietary intake of:

   A. Vitamin C.
   B. Folate.
   C. Potassium.
   D. Sodium.

5. Which hormone is secreted by the corpus luteum and adrenal glands and is responsible for changes in uterine endometrium in the second half of the menstrual cycle?

   A. Testosterone
   B. Estrogen
   C. Oxytocin
   D. Progesterone

6. Which contraceptive agent acts by suppressing release of the pituitary hormones FSH and LH, thus preventing ovulation?

   A. Progestin only
   B. Estrogen-progestin combination
   C. Mifeprex
   D. Ovral

7. When taking a health history from a female patient, the health care practitioner should report to the physician that which of these health problems would be a contraindication for prescribing an estrogen product?

   A. Osteoarthritis
   B. GERD
   C. Osteoporosis
   D. Liver disease

8. A young woman who is breast-feeding asks about an oral contraceptive that would be safe for her infant. Which type of oral contraceptive would not have an effect on lactation or nursing infant?

   A. Estrogen-progestin
   B. Biphasic preparation
   C. Progestin-only
   D. Triphasic preparation

9. A intrauterine device (IUD), Mirena, contains a reservoir of levonorgestrel, which is:

   A. Mifepristone.
   B. Synthetic progestin.
   C. Androgen/estrogen combination.
   D. Estrogen/progesterone combination.

10. Which hormone secreted by the posterior pituitary lobe stimulates the uterus to contract for childbirth then acts on the mammary gland to stimulate the release of milk?

    A. Testosterone
    B. Estrogen
    C. Oxytocin
    D. Progesterone

11. Which medication is used for preterm labor because its sympathomimetic action inhibits uterine contractions?

    A. Prostaglandin E_2
    B. Terbutaline
    C. Magnesium sulfate
    D. Oxytocin

12. Which medication is used for induction of labor with at-term or near-term pregnancies associated with hypertension, maternal diabetes, or uterine fetal death at term?

    A. Prostaglandin E_2
    B. Terbutaline
    C. Magnesium sulfate
    D. Oxytocin

13. Which medication is used for prevention and treatment of postpartum and postabortion hemorrhage?

    A. Oxytocin
    B. Methylergonovine
    C. Prostaglandin E_2
    D. Magnesium sulfate

14. Which medication is used for severe pre-eclampsia or eclampsia to control or prevent seizures by depressing the CNS and blocking neuromuscular transmission?

    A. Magnesium sulfate
    B. Dinoprostone
    C. Terbutaline
    D. Methylergonovine

15. Which of these medications is used for therapeutic abortions in the second trimester of pregnancy and/or uterine evacuation in cases of fetal death or congenital abnormalities incompatible with life?

    A. Prostaglandin E_2
    B. Terbutaline
    C. Methylergonovine
    D. Oxytocin

16. Administration of which of these medications requires constant maternal and fetal monitoring to prevent dangerous side effects such as uterine rupture or fetal trauma?

    A. Terbutaline
    B. Magnesium sulfate
    C. Methylergonovine
    D. Oxytocin

17. Which of these medications must be administered by a trained physician in a hospital where intensive care and surgical facilities are available because of the risk for severe side effects including respiratory and cardiac complications?

    A. Methylergonovine
    B. Terbutaline
    C. Prostaglandin E_2
    D. Lupron

18. Which of these medications are GnRH analogs that inhibit gonadotropin secretions and are used in the treatment of endometriosis?

    A. Terbutaline and Methergine
    B. Cervidil and Prepidil
    C. Cytotec and Pitocin
    D. Synarel and Lupron

Matching

Match the trade name of the reproductive system drugs listed in Column A with the generic name listed in Column B.

COLUMN A	COLUMN B
_____ 1. Megace	A. Sildenafil
_____ 2. Estrace	B. Danazol
_____ 3. Premphase, Prempro	C. Conjugated estrogens
_____ 4. Depo-Provera	D. Methyltestosterone
_____ 5. Menest	E. Megestrol acetate
_____ 6. Premarin	F. methyltestosterone with estrogens
_____ 7. Android, Testred	G. Vardenafil
_____ 8. CombiPatch	H. Esterified estrogens
_____ 9. Mifeprex	I. Medroxyprogesterone
_____ 10. Depo-Testosterone	J. Tadalafil
_____ 11. Estratest	K. Estradiol
_____ 12. Viagra	L. Conjugated estrogen/medroxyprogesterone
_____ 13. Cialis	M. Estradiol/Norethindrone
_____ 14. Levitra	N. Estrogen/progestin (postcoital contraception)

_____ 15. Syrarel

_____ 16. Lupron Depot

O. Mifepristone

P. Testosterone

Q. Nafarelin acetate

R. Leuprolide acetate

True or False

Circle T for true or F for false after reading each of the following statements.

1. T F When androgen therapy is used, anxiety, depression, and acne are some of the side effects that patients experience.

2. T F Patients taking androgens should be instructed to report any edema, jaundice, nausea, or vomiting to the physician.

3. T F Estrogens delivered in skin patches are released directly into the blood stream, bypassing the liver completely.

4. T F Estrogen therapy in the form of low-dose vaginal cream is used to treat atrophic vaginitis from decreased secretions.

5. T F Estrogen therapy can be used for postcoital contraception after rape or incest and to terminate pregnancy.

6. T F With estrogen therapy there is an increased risk of gallbladder disease.

7. T F Current medical recommendations for patients who need estrogen therapy is that combined estrogen-progestin therapy should not be used for prevention of cardiovascular disease.

8. T F Patients receiving progestins have the risk of edema and weight gain, and with prolonged use the risk of decreased bone density.

9. T F Progestins are used to treat threatened abortion during pregnancy although there is a risk of a potential adverse effect on the fetus.

10. T F Estrogens should be discontinued 4 weeks before a surgical procedure if possible.

11. T F Patients taking oral contraceptives may experience side effects such as fluid retention and changes in libido.

12. T F Estrogen products are absolutely contraindicated in a patient with a history of CVA, liver disease, or thrombophlebitis.

13. T F Postcoital contraception must be administered within 84 hours of unprotected intercourse.

14. T F The GnRH analog Lupron is administered monthly as an IM injection for at least 2 years.

15. T F The GnRH analog Synarel is administered as a nasal spray and treatment is limited to 6 months because prolonged use creates a hypoestrogenic state.

Case Study

Casey Tucker is a 27-year-old patient who is visiting the family planning clinic for the first time. Casey and her husband have two children but financial constraints make it necessary to limit future pregnancies. The health care practitioner who interviews Casey asks what she knows about oral contraceptive medications. Casey has never used contraceptive drugs before and wants to know how they work.

1. Which explanation should the health care practitioner provide?

A. They act by suppressing release of hormones that control ovulation.
B. They alter libido.
C. They decrease the thickness of cervical mucus.
D. They inhibit sperm motility.

2. The health care provider reviews Casey's health history, and finds that she has no history of thrombophlebitis or hypertension and is taking only over-the-counter medication such as acetaminophen (Tylenol). These data are important because

   A. Estrogens can cause these conditions to develop.
   B. Estrogens are contraindicated for patients who have either or both of these conditions.
   C. Contraceptives can interact adversely with acetaminophen.
   D. Contraceptives have many adverse side effects.

3. The physician prescribes Ortho-Novum, a monophasic estrogren progestin oral contraceptive. The health care practitioner should explain to Casey that this preparation may cause side effects such as

   A. Depression anxiety
   B. Increased menstrual flow
   C. Fluid retention and increased breast tenderness
   D. Nausea

4. What additional instruction should the health care practitioner give to Casey about her prescribed medication?

   A. Take it every morning with breakfast
   B. Take it every other day if side effects occur
   C. Stop taking it if any side effects occur
   D. Take it at dinner or bedtime, the same time every day

CHAPTER 25

Cardiovascular Drugs

Fill-in-the-Blank

Fill in the blank for each of the following statements.

1. Cardiac glycosides act directly on the heart muscle to _____ the strength of myocardial contractions.

2. Cardiac glycosides are used primarily in the treatment of _____ _____ _____ (CHF) to decrease pulmonary and systemic congestion by increasing the force of cardiac contractions and increasing cardiac output.

3. The process of establishing the correct therapeutic dose of digitalis for maintaining optimal functioning of the heart without toxic effects is called _____.

4. Serum digoxin levels are required to determine the therapeutic _____ dose.

5. The health care practitioner will always check the patient's _____ _____ prior to administering digoxin and document on the medication administration record.

6. When the patient's apical pulse rate is less than _____ beats per minutes, the health care practitioner should hold the digoxin until the physician is consulted.

7. Digoxin is available in tablet form, elixir or IV therapy and _____ adjustments may be required when changing from one form to another.

8. Early signs of digoxin toxicity are _____, nausea, and vomiting.

9. In the older adult, digoxin toxicity may be manifested by insomnia, _____, and mental disorders.

10. The health care practitioner assessing a patient receiving digoxin must always be aware of the patient's most recent serum potassium level, assessing for either _____ or _____.

11. Beta-adrenergic blocking agents inhibit sympathetic (adrenergic) nerve receptors, which cause a _____ in the blood pressure and pulse rate.

12. Hypotension in patients taking a beta-blocker is potentiated when the patient also takes a _____, another antihypertensive drug, muscle relaxants, sedatives, or alcohol.

13. Effectively dealing with hypertension through aggressive treatment is important since high blood pressure increases the risk of angina, myocardial infarction, heart failure, _____, and kidney disease.

14. The health care practitioner should teach patients taking an antiarrhythmic or an antihypertensive medication to always rise _____ from a reclining position.

15. Most patients who have hypertension meeting the criteria for drug therapy should be started on _____-type diuretics, either alone or in combination with a medication from another drug class.

16. For hypertensive patients with diabetes or high coronary disease risk, an initial therapy option is prescribing _____ _____ _____ such as nifedipine (Procardia) and diltiazem (Cardizem).

17. Medications such as atenolol (Tenormin) and propranolol (Inderal) are _____ _____ and can be used as initial therapy or for hypertensive patients with angina, postmyocardial infarction, and certain arrhythmias.

18. Patients taking calcium channel blockers should be taught to take the medication with a full glass of water on an empty stomach, one hour before or two hours after meals, to increase _____.

19. Pain from angina pectoris results from ischemia, insufficient blood supply, in the heart muscle due to obstruction or constriction of the _____ _____.

20. The treatment and prophylactic management of angina pectoris includes coronary _____ such as nitrates, beta-blockers, and calcium channel blockers.

21. The administration of vasodilators to patients who have angina dilates coronary arteries decreases myocardial _____ demand, stopping or reducing attacks of angina.

22. A sublingual tablet of _____ can be administered at the first sign of acute angina pectoris; if pain is not relieved, additional tablets can be administered at 5-minute intervals, with no more than three doses given in a 15-minute period.

23. Isosorbide, a nitrate used for long-term prophylactic management of angina pectoris, should be administered with a 12–14 hour nitrate-free interval between the last dose of the day and the first dose of the following day to reduce the risk of nitrate _____.

24. Another form of nitroglycerin is frequently applied as a _____ system and is used for long-term prophylactic management of angina pectoris.

25. The primary target of treatment in clinical lipid management is lowering _____ _____ lipoproteins, which carry the largest amount of the cholesterol in the blood and are in charge of transporting and depositing the cholesterol in arterial walls.

26. The health care practitioner must explain to patients taking statins to lower cholesterol that periodic blood tests are necessary to assess for elevated _____ enzymes.

27. Levophed administered IV is an adrenergic vasoconstrictor that increases systolic and diastolic blood pressure that is used only short term in the treatment of _____.

28. Anticoagulants interfere with the _____ process, they do not dissolve clots.

29. Although the purpose of the two classes of anticoagulants, warfarin and heparins, is the same, their actions are very _____.

30. Warfarin is administered _____ and has a slower onset of action than that of heparins; therefore, it is used for follow-up and long-term anticoagulant therapy.

31. Warfarin alters the synthesis of blood coagulation factors in the liver by interfering with the action of _____ _____.

32. International Normalized Ratio (INR) is the most commonly used laboratory method of monitoring therapy with _____ _____ and the results serve as the guide to determining dosage.

33. There are many drugs that interact with warfarin so it is important for the health care practitioner to check the patient's _____ medications before advising a patient about drug interactions.

34. Platelet inhibitors are used to provide _____ prevention in patients with a history of recent stroke, myocardial infarction, or established peripheral vascular disease.

35. Epoetin alfa (Epogen or Procrit) stimulates the bone marrow to produce more _____ _____ _____ and is approved for treatment of anemia in chronic renal failure, HIV infection, and anemia associated with chemotherapy.

36. Bleeding is the most serious complication of _____ therapy and can manifest as minor bleeding or major internal bleeding.

Multiple Choice

Circle the letter that best answers the question.

1. Which of these antiarrhythmic agents, while having the potential to lower blood pressure and slow the heartbeat, may cause tachycardia?

   A. Inderal and Tenormin
   B. Calan and Tenormin
   C. Quinidine and procainamide
   D. Procainamide and Inderal

2. The health care practitioner should assess patients taking any antiarrhythmic agent for which of these side effects?

   A. Hypertension and tachycardia
   B. Bradycardia and hypotension
   C. Elevated temperature
   D. Depressed respirations

3. Which of these types of antiarrhythmic agents counteract arrhythmias by suppressing the action of calcium in contraction of the heart muscle, reducing cardiac excitability and dilating the main coronary arteries?

   A. Adrenergic blockers
   B. Anticholinergics
   C. Beta-blockers
   D. Calcium channel blockers

4. The health care practitioner will instruct the patient taking a calcium channel blocker to be careful to avoid:

   A. Stool softeners and high fiber foods.
   B. Mild exercise.
   C. Taking this medication with grapefruit juice.
   D. Drinking large amounts of water.

5. Which of these antiarrhythmic agents combats arrhythmias by inhibiting sympathetic nerve receptors?

   A. Lidocaine
   B. Inderal
   C. Calan
   D. Quinidine

6. Which of these antiarrhythmic agents is typically administered as prophylactic therapy to maintain normal rhythm after the patient's rhythm has been converted by other methods?

   A. IA procainamide
   B. Xylocaine
   C. Lanoxin
   D. Tenormin

7. Syncope and tachycardia are side effects of which of these medications?

   A. Norvasc and Procardia XL
   B. Procainamide and quinidine
   C. Digoxin and Inderal
   D. Metoprolol and Tenormin

8. Which of these medications is contraindicated in a patient with congestive heart failure?

   A. Procainamide
   B. Digoxin
   C. Hydralazine
   D. Metoprolol

9. When administering the cardiac drug digoxin with an antiarrhythmic such as quinidine, the health care practitioner should observe the patient for signs of:

   A. Kidney failure
   B. Digoxin toxicity
   C. Liver failure
   D. Extensive skin rash

10. Which of these antihypertensive medications is a peripheral vasodilator that can be used to treat moderate-to-severe hypertension, particularly in patients with congestive heart failure?

    A. Prazosin
    B. Hydralazine
    C. Clonidine
    D. Valsartan

11. When a patient meets the criteria for drug therapy for hypertension, the first type of drug physicians typically order is usually:

    A. A thiazide diuretic.
    B. An antiarrhythmic.
    C. A peripheral vasodilator.
    D. An angiotensin receptor blocker.

12. Which of these categories of antihypertensives lower blood pressure by inhibiting the production of angiotensin II (a potent vasoconstrictor) with no resultant changes in heart rate or cardiac output?

    A. Thiazide diuretics
    B. Calcium channel blockers
    C. Beta-adrenergic blockers
    D. ACE inhibitors

13. Which of these types of antihypertensive drugs is a good choice for patients who have nephropathy, heart failure, diabetes, and cerebrovascular disease?

    A. Angiotensin-converting enzyme inhibitors
    B. Vasodilators
    C. Angiotensin receptor blockers
    D. Antiadrenergic agents

14. Which of these medications used for hypertension has been used successfully with patients experiencing opiate/nicotine withdrawal, vascular headaches, glaucoma, and severe pain in cancer patients?

    A. Prazosin
    B. Diltiazem
    C. Clonidine
    D. Valsartan

15. Which of these medications for angina pectoris which works to relieve acute chest pain associated with myocardial ischemia is available in sublingual tabs, sublingual spray, and IV, premixed or solution for injection?

    A. Metoprolol
    B. Nitroglycerin
    C. Isosorbide mononitrite
    D. Isosorbide dinitrate

16. When a health care practitioner administers topical nitroglycerin to a patient, which of these actions is essential?

    A. Apply the medication over any hairy skin area.
    B. Use the same site when applying the medication.
    C. Avoid touching the ointment or the inside of the transdermal patch.
    D. Apply the medication every 24 hours.

17. The health care practitioner should teach patients taking fast-acting nitrates to sit during administration to avoid falling in case of:

    A. Postural hypotension and syncope.
    B. Nausea and vomiting.
    C. Hypoglycemia.
    D. Loss of consciousness.

18. Which of these medications should not be used with nitrates because of the interaction between the two medications may possibly result in large, sudden, dangerous, drop in blood pressure?

    A. Allopurinol
    B. Aciphex
    C. Nexium
    D. Phosphodiesterase inhibitors

19. For long-term prophylactic treatment of angina pectoris, which of these types of oral medications are frequently prescribed?

    A. ACE inhibitors
    B. Nitroglycerin
    C. Phosphodiesterase inhibitors
    D. Beta blockers and calcium channel blockers

20. Which of these lipid-lowering medications are the most potent available for monotherapy and are considered the first choice in managing high cholesterol?

    A. Bile acid sequestrants
    B. Nicotinic acid (Niacin)
    C. Statins
    D. Cholesterol absorption inhibitors

21. Which of these side effects of bile acid sequestrants occur frequently and often affect the patient's compliance?

    A. Myalgia and muscle weakness
    B. Skin flushing, itching, and irritation
    C. Cholelithiasis, jaundice, and blood dyscracias
    D. Constipation, heartburn, nausea, and bloating

22. When a patient is taking bile acid sequestrants, the health care practitioner should teach the patient that

    A. Antibiotics, cardiac glycosides, fat-soluble vitamins, thiazide diuretics, and thyroid hormones should be taken at least 1 hour before or 4 hours after the bile acid sequestrant.
    B. The effects of oral anticoagulants and hypoglycemic agents are potentiated and the risk of serious muscle problems increases when bile acid sequestrants are taken with statins.
    C. When bile acid sequestrants are given with antihypertensives and vasodilators, the hypotensive effects are potentiated and loss of blood glucose control occurs when given with antidiabetic agents.
    D. There is an increased risk of myopathy and renal failure when bile acid sequestrants are administered with immunosuppressive drugs, erythromycin, and some antifungals.

23. Which of these side effects of immediate release preparations of nicotinic acid (niacin) that can be troublesome for the patient?

    A. Myalgia and muscle weakness
    B. Skin flushing, itching, and irritation
    C. Cholelithiasis, jaundice, and blood dyscracias
    D. Constipation, heartburn, nausea, and bloating

24. The health care practitioner should recognize that which of these interactions may occur when a patient is taking nicotinic acid (niacin)?

    A. Antibiotics, cardiac glycosides, fat-soluble vitamins, thiazide diuretics, and thyroid hormones should be taken at least 1 hour before or 4 hours after.
    B. The effects of oral anticoagulants and hypoglycemic agents are potentiated and the risk of serious muscle problems increases when taken with statins.
    C. When given with antihypertensives and vasodilators the hypotensive effects are potentiated and loss of blood glucose control occurs when given with antidiabetic agents.
    D. Increased risk of myopathy and renal failure when administered with immunosuppressive drugs, erythromycin, and some antifungals.

25. Side effects of the fibrates such as Tricor and Lopid that are effective in lowering triglyceride levels include:

    A. Myalgia and muscle weakness
    B. Skin flushing, itching, and irritation
    C. Cholelithiasis, jaundice, and blood dyscracias
    D. Constipation, heartburn, nausea, and bloating

26. The health care practitioner should teach patients who are taking administering ezetimibe (Zetia) that the drug should be administered at least:

    A. 1 hour before or 2 hours after administering antacids.
    B. 1 hour before administering fat-soluble vitamins and thyroid hormones.
    C. 4 hours between when also administering a statin drug.
    D. Every 4 hours while awake.

27. Enoxaparin (Lovenox) was the first low molecular weight heparin to be approved for:

    A. Prevention of deep vein thrombosis (DVT) in patients undergoing hip or knee replacement or abdominal surgery.
    B. Outpatient treatment of pulmonary embolism.
    C. Prophylactic treatment of angina.
    D. Inpatient treatment of acute pulmonary edema.

28. Patients with established peripheral vascular disease or a history of recent stroke or MI are typically prescribed prophylactic therapy consisting of:

    A. An oral anticoagulant.
    B. A platelet inhibitor.
    C. Nitrate coronary artery dilator.
    D. Low molecular dose heparin.

29. Which of these types of medication are used within the first few hours following a cerebrovascular accident or acute myocardial infarction to dissolve clots?

    A. Platelet inhibitors
    B. Anticoagulants
    C. Thrombolytic agents
    D. Colony-stimulating factors

30. Which of these medications are used to stimulate the bone marrow to produce more red blood cells?

    A. Platelet inhibitors
    B. Anticoagulants
    C. Thrombolytic agents
    D. Colony-stimulating factors

31. Thrombolytic therapy potentiates the body's process of fibrinolysis and reduces mortality after acute myocardial infarction (MI) or cerebral vascular accident (CVA) when used within the first:

    A. Hour after the patient is admitted to the hospital.
    B. 2 hours after the patient is admitted to the hospital.
    C. 6 hours after the incident occurred.
    D. 12 hours after the incident occurred.

32. Which of these agents has lessened the severity of mylosuppression in cancer patients and allowed chemotherapy doses to be intensified while allowing dose intensity to be maintained?

    A. Filgrastim (Neupogen)
    B. Epoetin (Procrit)
    C. Dipyridamole (Persantine)
    D. Alteplase (Activase)

Matching A

Match the trade name of the cardiac glycoside and antiarrhythmic drug listed in Column A with the generic name in Column B.

Column A	Column B
_____ 1. Rythmol	A. Propranolol
_____ 2. Calan	B. Atenolol
____ 3. Tenormin	C. Propafenone
_____ 4. Lanoxin, Lanoxicaps	D. Lidocaine
_____ 5. Inderal	E. Amiodarone
_____ 6. Xylocaine	F. Verapamil
_____ 7. Cordarone	G. Digoxin

Matching B

Match the antihypertensive drug listed in Column A with its category listed in Column B. Note that the choices in Column B can be used more than once.

COLUMN A	COLUMN B
_____ 1. Lisinopril (Zestril)	A. Beta-adrenergic blockers
_____ 2. Verapamil (Calan SR)	B. ACE inhibitors
____ 3. Atenolol (Tenormin)	C. Calcium channel blockers
_____ 4. Losartan (Cozaar)	D. Angiotensin receptor blockers
_____ 5. Ramipril (Altace)	E. Other antihypertensives
_____ 6. Valsartan (Diovan)	F. Thiazide diuretic
_____ 7. Hydrochlorothiazide	
_____ 8. Enalapril (Vasotec)	
_____ 9. Clonidine (Catapres)	
_____ 10. Captopril (Capoten)	
_____ 11. Prazosin (Minipres)	
_____ 12. Diltiazem (Cardizem LA)	
_____ 13. Methyldopa	
_____ 14. Carvedilol (Coreg)	
_____ 15. Nifedipine (Procardia XL)	

_____ 16. Benazepril (Lotensin)

_____ 17. Amiodipine (Norvasc)

_____ 18. Metoprolol (Lopressor)

Matching C

Match the coronary vasodilators and antilipemic agents listed in Column A with the action or use of the drug listed in Column B. Note that the choices in Column B can be used more than once.

COLUMN A	**COLUMN B**
_____ 1. Atorvastatin (Lipitor)	A. Lovastatin/niacin
_____ 2. Colesevelam	B. Inhibits the release of free fatty acids from adipose tissue, decreases hepatic lipoprotein synthesis (nicotinic acid)
_____ 3. Isorbide dinitrate tabs PO	
_____ 4. Vytorin	C. Ezetimibe/simvastatin
_____ 5. Simvastatin (Zocor)	D. Inhibits intestinal absorption of both dietary and biliary cholesterol, blocking its transport in the small intestine (cholesterol absorption inhibitor)
_____ 6. Nitrotstat tabs S.L.	
_____ 7. Advicor	E. Especially effective in patients who have extremely high triglyceride levels (fibric acid derivatives)
_____ 8. Ezetimibe (Zetia)	
_____ 9. Niacin (Niaspan, Slo-Niacin)	F. Absorbs and comes together with bile acids to form an insoluble complex to facilitate its excretion through feces (bile acid sequestrants)
_____ 10. Isosorbide mononitrate [Imdur (SR)]	
_____ 11. Fenofibrate (Tricor)	G. Inhibit the enzyme for cholesterol synthesis (statins)
_____ 12. Nitro-Dur	H. Dilates coronary arteries; reduces cardiac oxygen demand (prophylactic antianginal nitrate)
	I. Dilates coronary arteries and improves blood flow to heart muscle (fast-acting nitrate)

Matching D

Match the medication listed in Column A with the class of the drug listed in Column B. Note that the choices in Column B can be used more than once.

COLUMN A	**COLUMN B**
_____ 1. Filgrastim (Neupogen)	A. Warfarin (anticoagulant)
_____ 2. Epoetin alfa (Epogen)	B. Unfractionated heparin (anticoagulant)
_____ 3. Dalteparin (Fragmin)	C. Low-molecular weight heparins (anticoagulant)
_____ 4. Warfarin (Coumadin)	D. Platelet inhibitors
_____ 5. Enoxaparin (Lovenox)	E. Thrombolytic agents
_____ 6. Streptokinase (Kabikinase)	F. Colony-stimulating factors
_____ 7. Aspirin (Ecotrin, Ascriptin)	
_____ 8. Alteplase, TPA (Activase)	
_____ 9. Clopidogrel (Plavix)	
_____ 10. Dipyridamole with aspirin (Aggrenox)	
_____ 11. IV or SQ Heparin	

True or False

Circle T for true or F for false after reading each of the following statements.

1. T F The health care practitioner should advise the patient to discontinue the digoxin immediately when digoxin toxicity is confirmed.

2. T F Any patient whose medication regime includes antacids, neomycin, rifampin, and digoxin should take the digoxin at a different time than the other medications to avoid an unwanted interaction.

3. T F Patients taking Inderal or Tenormin are at risk for bronchospasm, especially if they have a history of asthma.

4. T F Diabetic patients taking beta-adrenergic blocking agents should be extremely cautious since the beta-blocker may cause hypoglycemia and the typical tachycardic response to hypoglycemia is blocked.

5. T F Quinidine is an antiarrhythmic medication with numerous and possibly life-threatening side effects.

6. T F Hyperglycemia, hypertension, tachycardia, and tinnitus are possible side effects of quinidine.

7. T F A side effect of the antihypertensive methyldopa (Aldomet) is sexual dysfunction.

8. T F Patients with prehypertension are encouraged to reduce weight if overweight or obese and to use the DASH eating plan.

9. T F DASH stands for "dietary approaches to stop hypertension" and includes an eating plan with sodium reduction, increased physical activity, modified alcohol use, and smoking cessation.

10. T F The health care practitioner should caution patients about not skipping or doubling a dose of an antiarrhythmic and never to discontinue the drug without consulting their physician.

11. T F Patients taking calcium channel blockers should be taught to avoid grapefruit juice because it can increase the risk of hypotension and other adverse effects.

12. T F Antihypertensives are not a cure for hypertension, they only control it; if the antihypertensive medication is abruptly withdrawn, rebound hypertension can occur.

13. T F Isosorbide is available in SQ and IM injections that can be administered once daily for prevention of chest pain from angina pectoris.

14. T F Nitroglycerin tablets should be stored away from heat and in a glass bottle with a tightly fitting metal screw top.

15. T F The antidote for serious bleeding complications in patients on warfarin therapy is protamine sulfate.

16. T F Thrombolytic therapy is used for prophylaxis for patients with a history of stroke, recent MI, or established peripheral vascular disease.

17. T F The tolerability of the platelet inhibitor clopidogrel (Plavix) is similar to aspirin, but it is less likely to cause gastrointestinal bleeding.

Case Study

Roger Taper, a 63-year-old man, is diagnosed with a DVT, and he has a history of congestive heart failure. He has been hospitalized to receive anticoagulant therapy. His physician is planning for Roger's discharge, where he will take a PO anticoagulant and a low-molecular weight heparin (LMWH) to continue his treatment at home.

1. Mr. Taper asks the health care practitioner why heparin is important and why it cannot be taken by mouth. Which of these responses would be correct?

   A. Heparin acts to inhibit the action of fibrin in clot formation to prevent another clot, but it is not absorbed from the GI tract.
   B. Heparin can be administered by mouth but acts more quickly by the IV or subcutaneous routes.
   C. Heparin alters the synthesis of blood coagulation factors in the liver by interfering with vitamin K, and it cannot be absorbed through the GI tract.
   D. Heparin acts in the liver to inhibit the action of fibrin in clot formation, thus stopping additional clot formation, and it is not absorbed as rapidly when given by mouth.

2. The health care practitioner explains that LMWH has a better bioavailability and produces more predictable anticoagulant response than which of these?

   A. Thrombolytic agents
   B. Platelet inhibitors
   C. Unfractioned type of heparin
   D. Antilipemic agents

3. The health care practitioner administering heparin is aware that the antidote for serious bleeding complications during heparin therapy is:

   A. Vitamin K.
   B. Protamine sulfate.
   C. Enoxaparin.
   D. Salicylate.

4. When teaching the patient to administer the injections of Lovenox at home, the health care practitioner should stress which of these to the patient?

   A. Give the injection in the deltoid muscle twice a day for 1 week.
   B. Rub site briskly with alcohol to increase blood flow to the area to be injected.
   C. Aspirate and then administer the heparin slowly into the fat pad of the upper arm.
   D. Administer the heparin slowly SQ into the fat pad along the lower abdomen.

5. The health care practitioner explains to Mr. Taper about regulation of medication dosage, the lab work to monitor anticoagulation therapy. Which explanation is correct?

   A. Monitoring of the anticoagulant effect of LMWH is not necessary, and the International Normalized Radio (INR) guides dosages of Coumadin.
   B. The partial prothrombin time (PTT) will be drawn weekly after discharge to evaluate the effects of the LMWH, and the Coumadin dosages will be adjusted as needed.
   C. Coumadin will be monitored by the PTT and the LMWH will be monitored by the INR.
   D. There is no lab work needed; the patient will be taught about side effects and problems associated with anticoagulation and when to contact the physician.

6. The health care practitioner should teach the patient his responsibility while on anticoagulation therapy is to

   A. Careful observe skin, gums, urine, and stools daily and immediately report of any signs of bleeding
   B. Cut back on participation in contact sports
   C. Use a non-electric razor
   D. Eat plenty of foods rich in vitamin D

CHAPTER 26

Respiratory System Drugs and Antihistamines

Fill-in-the-Blank

Fill in the blank for each of the following statements.

1. Oxygen is administered to patients for _____ (insufficient oxygen supply to tissues) via nasal cannula, masks, tents, and hoods.

2. Patients who have chronic obstructive pulmonary disease (COPD) may respond to prolonged oxygen at high _____ with hypoventilation or apnea.

3. Premature infants who are exposed to high concentrations of oxygen for prolonged periods of time may develop _____.

4. Oxygen is not flammable but it does support _____; therefore, anything that may spark such as smoking, matches, or electrical equipment is not allowed in rooms where oxygen is in use.

5. Caffeine citrate, a respiratory _____, is used for the treatment of neonatal apnea.

6. In the treatment of hyperventilation or hiccups, inhalation of _____ _____, which is a respiratory stimulant, improves rate and depth of respirations.

7. Acute respiratory conditions such as asthma require bronchodilators to relax the smooth muscles of the bronchial tree, relieve _____ and improve vital capacity of the lungs.

8. Sympathomimetics (adrenergics) are potent bronchodilators but also affect the entire sympathetic nervous system and can cause cardiac irregularities, _____ and hyperglycemia.

9. The inhalation route is preferred for the sympathomimetic bronchodilators because systemic adverse _____ are minimized.

10. Inhalers that provide medication only under the pressure of the patient's inhalation rather than through compression of the valve are called "_____ _____ Inhalers."

11. Anticholinergics block the parasympathetic response and achieve bronchodilation by decreasing the _____ that promotes bronchospasm.

12. Health care practitioners should teach patients taking anticholinergics to maintain adequate _____ to avoid mucus plugging that occludes the airway.

13. Tiotropium (Spiriva) is structurally similar to ipratropium (Atrovent) and can be administered _____.

14. Xanthines can be administered for acute episodes of asthma but are no longer a _____ _____ treatment because of modest clinical effectiveness, need for serum monitoring, and many adverse effects and drug interactions.

15. Xanthines are usually administered with sustained release formulations with other respiratory system drugs such as adrenergics and _____.

16. The health care practitioner should teach the patient using inhaled corticosteroids to rinse the mouth after using the inhaler to avoid oral _____ infections.

17. The health care practitioner should explain the correct method of administering inhaled bronchodilators and corticosteroids to the patient is to administer the _____ before the _____.

18. For patients who have asthma, COPD, and those who are prone to addiction, _____ antitussives are contraindicated.

19. Patients with COPD, asthma, cardiovascular disorders, benign prostatic hypertrophy, and seizure disorders should be instructed to avoid self-medicating with antihistamines without the specific _____ of the physician.

20. Diphenhydramine (Benadryl) is used in the treatment of _____ to combat the increased capillary permeability, edema, inflammation, and itching.

21. The leading cause of preventable disease and death in the United States is _____ _____.

Multiple Choice

Circle the letter that best answers the question.

1. Albuterol, epinephrine, and salmeterol are all rapid-acting bronchodilators of which classification?

   A. Corticosteroids
   B. Anticholinergics
   C. Sympathomimetics
   D. Xanthines

2. Theophylline is an example of which type of bronchodilator?

   A. Xanthines
   B. Anticholinergics
   C. Sympathomimetics
   D. Corticosteroids

3. Flovent is an example of which classification of respiratory medication?

   A. Anticholinergics
   B. Xanthines
   C. Sympathomimetics
   D. Corticosteroids

4. Zafirlukast (Accolate) and montelukast (Singulair), which primarily help to control the inflammatory process of asthma and help prevent asthma symptoms and attacks, are examples of which type of respiratory medication?

   A. Antileukotrienes
   B. Anticholinergics
   C. Sympathomimetics
   D. Corticosteroids

5. Cromolyn, used as a prophylactic management for individuals with asthma and in prevention of exercise-induced asthma, is an example of which type of respiratory medication?

   A. Antileukotriene
   B. Mast-cell stabilizer
   C. Sympathomimetic
   D. Corticosteroid

6. Acetylcysteine (Mucomyst) liquefies pulmonary secretions and is classified as which type of respiratory medication?

   A. Antihistamine
   B. Antitussive
   C. Mucolytic
   D. Expectorant

7. Guaifenesin, which increases secretions, reduces viscosity, and helps the patient expel sputum, is classified as which type of respiratory medication?

   A. Antihistamine
   B. Antitussive
   C. Mucolytic
   D. Expectorant

8. Codeine and hydrocodone are added to some cough syrups to prevent coughing in patients with a dry nonproductive cough. When these narcotics are used this way they are classified as:

   A. Antihistamines
   B. Antitussives
   C. Mucolytics
   D. Expectorants

9. Diphenhydramine (Benadryl), used in the treatment of allergies, as an adjunctive treatment for anaphylactic reaction after the acute symptoms are controlled, and in symptomatic treatment of vertigo, is classified as which type of respiratory medication?

   A. Antihistamine
   B. Decongestant
   C. Mucolytic
   D. Expectorant

10. Anticholinergic side effects of first-generation antihistamines include:

    A. Runny nose and urinary frequency
    B. Hypoventilation in the older adult and arrhythmias
    C. Hyperglycemia and urinary frequency
    D. Drying of the eyes and hypotension in the older adult

11. Phenylephrine (Neosynephrine) and pseudoephedrine (Sudafed) constrict blood vessels in the respiratory tract, resulting in shrinkage of swollen mucous membranes and are classified as which type of respiratory medication?

    A. Expectorants
    B. Antihistamines
    C. Decongestants
    D. Mucolytics

12. The health care practitioner should instruct patients with respiratory conditions taking respiratory system drugs to:

    A. Limit exercise to preserve respiratory function
    B. Avoid combining prescribed medications with other prescription or over-the-counter drugs or alcohol
    C. Limit the amount of water and fluids taken PO
    D. Avoid going outside, especially in cold weather

Matching A

Match the bronchodilator, corticosteroid, or asthma prophylaxis listed in Column A with the category or use of the drugs in listed in Column B. Note that the choices in Column B can be used more than once.

COLUMN A

_____ 1. Beclomethasone (QVAR, Beconase AQ)

_____ 2. Theophylline (Uniphyl)

_____ 3. Salmeterol (Serevent Diskus)

_____ 4. Cromolyn sodium

_____ 5. Tiotropium (Spriva)

_____ 6. Ipratropium bromide (Atrovent)

_____ 7. Budesonide (Pulmicort Respules)

_____ 8. Adrenalin

_____ 9. Ipratropium bromide/albuterol (Combivent, DuoNeb)

_____ 10. Montelukast (Singulair)

_____ 11. Ventolin HFA

_____ 12. Fluticasone (Flovent, Flonase)

_____ 13. Albuterol sulfate (Vospire ER)

_____ 14. Fluticasone with salmeterol (Advair Diskus)

_____ 15. Zafirlukast (Accolate)

_____ 16. Mometasone (Nasonex)

_____ 17. Levalbuterol (Xopenex)

_____ 18. Foridil Aerolizer

_____ 19. Triamcinolone (Nasacort AQ)

_____ 20. Theophylline

COLUMN B

A. Sympathomimetics (adrenergics)

B. Anticholinergics

C. Xanthines

D. Corticosteroids

E. Asthma prophylaxis

F. Corticosteroid/sympathomimetic

G. Anticholinergic/sympathomimetic

Matching B

Match the trade name listed in Column A with the generic name listed in Column B. Note that one of the choices in Column B can be used more than once.

COLUMN A

_____ 1. Chlor-Trimeton

_____ 2. Mucinex, Robitussin

_____ 3. Tavist Allergy

_____ 4. Sudafed, Efidac

_____ 5. Tessalon

_____ 6. Hycodan

_____ 7. Astelin

_____ 8. Cheratussin AC

COLUMN B

A. Pseudoephedrine

B. Clemastine (first generation)

C. Diphenhydramine

D. Desloratadine (second generation)

E. Azelastine

F. Fexofenadine (second generation)

G. Hydrocodone bitartrate

H. Cetrizine (second generation)

(Matching continued on next page)

COLUMN A (continued)	COLUMN B (continued)
____ 9. Zyrtec	I. Oxymetazoline
____ 10. Afrin	J. Loratadine (second generation)
____ 11. Hydromet	K. Benzonatate
____ 12. Mucomyst	L. Phenylephrine
____ 13. Benadryl, Diphenhist, Benadryl Allergy	M. Codeine/guaifenesin
____ 14. Clarinex	N. Chlorpheniramine (first generation)
____ 15. Robitussin-DM	O. Guaifenesin
____ 16. Allegra	P. Acetylcysterine (mucolytic)
____ 17. Neo-Synephrine, Nostril	Q. Dextromethorphan/guaifenesin
____ 18. Claritin, Alavert	R. Hydrocodone with homatropine

True or False

Circle T for true or F for false after reading each of the following statements.

1. T F Metered dose inhalers (MDIs) are frequently used and the use of a spacer or reservoir device assists in optimizing drug delivery within the lungs.

2. T F Theophylline is generally reserved for patients with COPD who do not respond to inhaled long-acting bronchodilators.

3. T F Xanthines have the possibility of causing GI distress, CNS stimulation, cardiac palpitations, and hyperglycemia.

4. T F Inhaled corticosteroids have more systemic side effects than oral or IV administration.

5. T F Zafirlukast (Accolate) can be used to treat an acute episode of asthma in a young child.

6. T F First-generation antihistamines and decongestants are contraindicated in patients with benign prostatic hypertrophy (BPH).

7. T F Second-generation antihistamines cause fewer anticholinergic effects than first-generation antihistamines.

8. T F Patients taking decongestants should be cautioned by the health care practitioner to use either nasal or oral decongestants for only a few days to avoid rebound congestion.

Case Study

Jay Rose, 45 years old, attends the medical clinic once every year. He has been smoking cigarettes for 25 years and expresses a desire to quit. He asks the health care practitioner in the clinic how he can quit smoking.

1. When discussing with Jay about smoking cessation, the health care practitioner explains that cessation aids are available to assist with the process, including which of these?

   A. Nicorette gum, Nicoderm CQ Patch, and the Nicotrol inhaler
   B. Methadone, antihistamines, and bronchodilators
   C. Use of an artificial "smoker"
   D. Zantac and other H2 blockers

2. The health care practitioner is aware that Jay may also need an antidepressant to help him through the withdrawal symptoms associated with smoking cessation. Which antidepressant has been found to be successful when used in combination with other aids for smoking cessation?

   A. Sertraline (Zoloft)
   B. Amitriptyline (Elavil)
   C. Bupropion (Wellbutrin)
   D. Citalopram (Celexa)

3. The health care practitioner explains there are side effects of smoking cessation aids containing nicotine, including:

   A. Cardiac irritability and insomnia.
   B. Constipation and pale skin color.
   C. Nausea, vomiting, and low blood pressure.
   D. Jaundice and decreased sweating.

4. The health care practitioner suggests to Jay that it would be beneficial in his smoking cessation to participate in which of these?

   A. Cardiac rehabilitation program.
   B. Group exercise program.
   C. Behavior modification program.
   D. Psychoanalysis of eating habits.

5. Jay should be instructed that when using the smoking cessation aids containing nicotine, he should:

   A. Use the aids for 1 week and then stop smoking completely.
   B. Smoke only seven cigarettes the day he starts and decrease by one each day.
   C. Smoke only four cigarettes per day for the first week, two each day for the second week, and then stop.
   D. Not smoke at all because the aid contains nicotine and he would be getting an overdose if he smoked cigarettes.

6. What additional information should the health care practitioner provide Jay about smoking cessation aids?

   A. Use the aids with caution if he has a history of allergies.
   B. Dental problems might be exacerbated by chewing gum and another aid should be chosen.
   C. Smoke one or two cigarettes if he is in a stressful situation.
   D. Use the cessation aid at bedtime to promote sleep.

CHAPTER 27

Drugs and Older Adults

Fill-in-the-Blank

Fill in the blank for each of the following statements.

1. The absorption process is affected by the aging body's _decrease_ gastric motility, increasing gastric pH.

2. Because aging is an individualized process, older adults need to realize that there are _____ changes in body composition and organ function which can affect reaction to drugs.

3. After drugs are absorbed, many of them attach to _____, the principal protein our bodies use to bind drugs.

4. The older adult has _less_ serum albumin levels and thus less protein available for binding and transporting drug molecules.

5. With less protein to bind with, more free, pharmacologically active drug reaches receptor sites and produce _greater_ than expected response.

6. Risks of side effects of medications are a greater concern to older adults who have conditions such as malnutrition, _diabetes_, cancer, surgery, burns, and liver disease when these patients take medications such as naproxen, phenytoin, and valproic acid (Depakote).

7. Older adults who are taking drugs that are water soluble, such as digoxin and lithium are at risk for adverse effects, which become _cumative_ over time.

8. Functional liver tissue and blood flow to the liver decline with age, resulting in the older adult's loss of ability to _____ or break down drugs; therefore, drugs remain in the body longer.

9. With decreased liver function, repeated dosing can cause the accumulation of the drug and increase the risk of _toxisity._.

10. Older adults who have illnesses such as hypertension, heart failure, and diabetes are at greater risk for developing toxic effects from prescribed drugs because drug by-products normally eliminated through the _____ can accumulate because of the decline in _____ function.

11. Repeated doses and slowed metabolism of long-acting _____ have been implicated in falls and hip fractures in older adults because of side effects such as daytime sedation, dizziness, lethargy, and ataxia.

12. Older adults are more likely to have adverse drug reactions to anticholinergics and drugs that product significant anticholinergic effects such as antidepressants, antiparkinson agents, antipsychotics, antispasmodics, and _antihystamine_.

13. The Beers Study, updated and revised in 2003, identifies medications that are potentially _inappropriay_ for older adults and is available for download free of charge.

14. The increase of anticholinergic drugs circulating in the system of older adults is often gradual and the consequences of a drug _overdose_ may not be recognized or considered to just to be due to aging.

15. Excessive use of drugs or prescriptions or many drugs used at one time by older adults is called _polypharmacy_.

Multiple Choice

Circle the letter that best answers the questions.

1. Which of these statements about the use of medications by older adults is true?

   A. Medication-related problems, such as cognitive impairment and behavior changes, are frequently the result of medication therapy in older adults.
   B. Responses to medication will remain basically the same one ages.
   C. Anticipate older adults' exact response to drug therapy and expect less adverse effects since their metabolism is slower.
   D. It is relatively easy to separate the effects of aging from the effects of disease processes or drug therapy responses.

2. What effect does decreased gastric motility have upon older adults' response to medications?

   A. Absorption is decreased
   B. Distribution is enhanced
   C. Metabolism is slowed
   D. Excretion is enhanced

3. Cumulative effects of drugs taken by older adults are related to which of these processes?

   A. Faster metabolism
   B. Impaired excretion
   C. The older adult's diet includes more foods that create production of acid in the stomach
   D. The gall bladder does not function as well in the older adult

4. Use of antacids by older adults affects absorption of medications such as quinolone antibiotics and tetracycline and these medications not be taken within what time period after the use of antacids?

   A. 30 minutes
   B. 1 hour
   C. 1½ hours
   D. 2 hours

5. In the older adult, taking drugs that are water soluble may result in higher plasma concentration and cause adverse reactions because the older adult has:

   A. Decreased total body water.
   B. Less functional liver mass.
   C. Decreased glomerular filtration rate.
   D. Decreased gastric motility.

6. Decreased kidney size, blood flow, and glomerular filtration result in a decline in creatinine clearance in the older adult. Which process of pharmacokinetics does this affect?

   A. Metabolism
   B. Distribution
   C. Excretion
   D. Absorption

7. Which of these sleeping medications are suggested for the older adult on a short-term or PRN basis?

   A. Restoril
   B. Atarax
   C. Zolpidem
   D. Dalmane

8. Warfarin (Coumadin) and aspirin are drugs highly protein-bound. In the older adult, plasma albumin levels typically drop, which affect the drug's:

   A. Absorption.
   B. Distribution.
   C. Metabolism.
   D. Excretion.

9. Which types of antihistamines are preferred for the older client?

   A. Phenergan or Atarax
   B. Benadryl or Chlor-Trimeton
   C. Any with anticholinergic effects
   D. Any nonanticholinergic antihistamines

10. Which SSRI antidepressant is not recommended for the older adult?

   A. Paxil
   B. Prozac
   C. Zoloft
   D. Celexa

Matching A

Match the drugs potentially inappropriate for the older adult (noninclusive) listed in Column A with the drug classification in Column B. Note that one of the choices in Column B can be used more than once.

COLUMN A	COLUMN B
_____ 1. Chlorpropamide (Diabinese)	A. Antidepressants
_____ 2. Ferrous sulphate	B. Short-acting benzodiazepines
_____ 3. Dicyclomine (Bentyl)	C. Long-acting benzodiazepines
_____ 4. Diazepam (Valium)	D. NSAIDs
_____ 5. Nitrofurantoin (Macrodantin)	E. Oral hypoglycemic
_____ 6. Meperidine (Demerol)	F. Analgesics
_____ 7. Haloperidol (Haldol)	G. Muscle relaxants
_____ 8. Hydroxyzine (Vistaril, Atarax)	H. Anti-infectives
_____ 9. Hyoscyamine (Cystospaz, Levsin, Levsinex)	I. Antispasmodics
_____ 10. Hydrochlorothiazide (Esidrix)	J. Iron
_____ 11. Alprazolam (Xanax)	K. Antiemetics
_____ 12. Amitriptyline (Elavil)	L. Antipsychotics
_____ 13. Ketorolac (Toradol)	M. Antihistamines
_____ 14. Methocarbamol (Robaxin)	N. Antihypertensives
_____ 15. Trimethobenzamide (Tigan)	

Matching B

Match the drugs potentially inappropriate for the older adult (noninclusive) listed in Column A with the drug classification in Column B. Note that the choices in Column B can be used more than once.

COLUMN A	COLUMN B
_____ 1. Promethazine (Phenergan)	A. Histamine 2 blocker
_____ 2. Belladonna alkaloids (Donnatal)	B. Decongestants
_____ 3. Propranolol (Inderal)	C. Platelet inhibitors
_____ 4. Lorazepam (Ativan)	D. Antihistamines
_____ 5. Fluoxetine (Prozac)	E. Antispasmodics

_____ 6. Doxepin (Sinequan)

_____ 7. Disopyramide (Norpace)

_____ 8. Clonidine (Catapres)

_____ 9. Dipyridamole (Persantine)

_____ 10. Pseudoephedrine (Sudafed)

_____ 11. Cimetidine (Tagamet)

F. Antiarrhythmics

G. Short-acting benzodiazepines

H. Antihypertensives

I. Antidepressants

True or False

Circle T for true or F for false after reading each of the following statements.

1. T F Older adults with hypertension, heart failure, and diabetes have an even further reduced creatinine clearance.

2. T F Nephrotoxic drugs, such as the aminoglycosides, can prove exceptionally dangerous for the older adult with reduced renal function.

3. T F Drugs such as Benadryl and Lopressor are among those which do not cause mental impairment in older adults.

4. T F Older adults are more likely to have adverse drug reactions to drugs that produce anticholinergic effects such as some antipsychotics, antidepressants, antispasmodics, and antihistamines.

5. T F Digoxin is a medication that the health care practitioner should monitor carefully for toxicity in the older adult because of slowed clearance from the system.

Case Study

Susan Marsh is a 65-year-old woman who has been diagnosed with arthritis and takes over-the-counter nonsteroidal anti-inflammatory drugs (NSAIDs) who comes to the clinic for a physical examination. She tells the health care practitioner that she takes other medications ordered by other physicians but did not bring them with her today.

1. Knowing that polypharmacy is a problem with many older adults, what should the health care practitioner encourage Susan to do?

   A. Bring the prescription drugs for the doctor to see at her next visit.
   B. Make a list of all her medications, prescribed or over the counter, vitamins, herbal remedies, and topical medications to keep in her wallet or purse, and send a copy to the physician as soon as possible.
   C. Ask a family member to remind her about her daily medications.
   D. Continue taking her NSAIDs and discontinue all other prescribed or over the counter medications.

2. Because NSAIDs can cause health problems in older adults, it is most important for the health care practitioner to assess Susan for

   A. Evidence of a "silent" gastrointestinal bleed
   B. Signs of tinnitus
   C. Signs of hypertension
   D. Signs of constipation, or diarrhea

3. The health care practitioner should review how Susan takes her NSAIDs. Which information is important to emphasize?

   A. Increase her fluid intake
   B. Take an additional dose if she is having pain
   C. Take the medications with food
   D. Limit her exercise to reduce pain

4. The health care practitioner should also ask Susan to avoid which of these while she is taking NSAIDs?

   A. Fresh fruits and vegetables
   B. Processed meat products
   C. Foods high in calcium
   D. Alcoholic beverages and aspirin

Notes

Notes

Notes

Notes

Notes

Notes